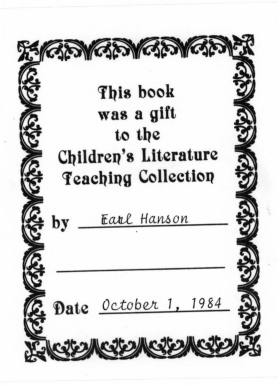

This book
was a gift
to the
Children's Literature
Teaching Collection

by *Earl Hanson*

_____

Date *October 1, 1984*

You Are Beautiful: You Really Are . . .

YOU ARE *Beautiful:*
YOU REALLY ARE . . .

by
Joyce Proctor Beaman

Part I—Internal Beauty
You Are A Special Someone . . .

Part II—External Beauty
You Are Not Just A Body—You Are Somebody

Part III—Eternal Beauty
The Ultimate Crowning

Webb-Newcomb Company, Inc. —*Publishers*
WILSON, NORTH CAROLINA 27893

You Are Beautiful:
You Really Are . . .

Printed in the United States of America
All Rights Reserved

Published by **Webb-Newcomb Company, Inc.** —*Publishers*

308 N. E. VANCE STREET
WILSON, NORTH CAROLINA 27893

Library of Congress Catalog Card Number: 81-52869
ISBN: 0-935054-06-5

THIS BOOK
IS DEDICATED
TO ALL THE BEAUTIFUL PEOPLE
WHO HAVE TOUCHED MY LIFE
AND WHO KEPT SAYING:
"JOYCE, PLEASE WRITE ANOTHER BOOK."

Because

Because of your strong faith, I kept the
   track
   Whose sharp-set stones my strength
   had well-nigh spent
I could not meet your eyes if I turned
   back;
   So on I went.

Because you would not yield belief in me
   The threatening crags that rose my way to bar,
I conquered inch by crumbling inch—to
   see
   The goal afar.

And though I struggle toward it through
   hard years,
   Or flinch, or falter blindly, yet within,
"You can!" unwavering my spirit hears
   And I shall win.

Author Unknown

TABLE OF CONTENTS

Part I . . . Internal Beauty . . . You Are
              A Special Someone 11

1. You Are Beautiful Even If You Are Not
   Aware of It 13
2. You Are Beautiful in Many Ways 17
3. Simplicity 21
4. Counting Good Things 24
5. A Positive Self-Image 28
6. Praise 32
7. Adjusting to Others 35
8. Love and the Family 38
9. Putting Sparkle in Your Eyes 45
10. The Art of Listening 51
11. Concerning Men 54
12. No More Trophies 56
13. Joy in Patriotism 58
14. Solving Problems: Over 40 Ways
    to Consider 64
15. What Is Really Important Anyway? 85

Part II . . . External Beauty . . .
              You Are Not Just a Body—
              You Are Somebody 89

16. The Pursuit of Excellence 91
17. Charm 95
18. What Is Class? 98
19. Serenity 103

20. Silence 107
21. The Voice 110
22. Putting One's Best Foot Forward 113
23. Things Not to Do If You Want to Be
    Appealing to the One You Love 115
24. The Face 118
25. Cosmetics 123
26. Beauty Aid Discoveries 128
27. Wardrobe-Clothes-You 132
28. The Essential Negatives 138
29. Manners 140
30. Visual Poise 143
31. Non-Verbal Communication 149
32. Using Time Wisely 151
33. Word Pronunciations and Practical
    Grammar 156
34. Exercise 166
35. Dieting: Heaps of Hints to Help 171
36. Nutrition 186
37. Stress: A Dozen Ways to Combat It 190

Part III . . . Eternal Beauty . . .
              The Ultimate Crowning 193

38. Reaching Beyond Ourselves 195
39. It Takes Only One 198
40. It Takes Only Five Minutes 201
41. Sometimes We Stand Alone 203
42. O, Lord, God, Help Us to Find Our Way . . . 206
43. Turning Aside to the Quiet Roads 209

44. Finding My Place Amid the Throng 212
45. Tarnished Trophies 214
46. What, Then, Is an Education? 216
47. If You Love Me, Tell My Mother 218
48. Daddy Does the Lights 221
49. Regrets 224
50. Dear God, Please Give Me One
    More Sunrise 227
51. Faith 229
52. One Solitary Life 231
53. Does She Think She Is Beautiful? 233
54. You Are Beautiful When You Walk
    with God 235

Index 236

Acknowledgements 238

Additional Acknowledgements 239

Further Acknowledgements 240

Part I

INTERNAL BEAUTY

You Are A Special Someone

Chapter 1

You Are Beautiful Even If You Are Not Aware of It

You are a special someone.

And you are beautiful, even if you do not know it or even if you are not aware of it. You may not have desired to be, or thought about being, or tried to be, but in some special way, you are beautiful — whether male or female, young or old. Your beauty may lie dormant or unpolished or unsurfaced, but it is there. By fingerprints and appearance, every person is different: no one is like you. Yet, there is another way, too, that we are different: there is a special beauty about you or within you.

When we think about beauty, we immediately think of Hollywood, the Miss America pageant, and the lovely celebrities of television and stage. Among other attributes, these people have physical beauty — and much of this book is concerned with physical beauty.

But there is beauty in you beyond physical beauty. It flows and shows in the things you do and say, in the things you stand for or stand against, in what you are inwardly as well as outwardly.

Yet, finding people who are completely satisfied with the way they look or live is almost impossible. The reply would be: "If it were not for my hair . . . or my weight . . . or my birthmark . . . or my large knees . . . or my depression . . . or my lack of faith." The list is endless, encompassing concerns for almost every part of life and every part of the body.

Three thoughts offer possible solutions:

1. Can I do anything to correct what I consider to be my imperfection?
2. Am I willing to take action?
3. If nothing can be done, do I have other qualities or attributes that cover or cloud completely what I consider to be a weakness or fault?

While I was talking with a friend about a superior administrator and his unique leadership, she replied: "His name sounds familiar. I may have had a class with him at the university. Is he bald? Does he wear glasses?"

I thought for a moment.

"I really do not remember," I said. "I shall have to check the next time I see him."

I was sincere. I really did not know whether he was bald or wore glasses. His personality and character were so outstanding that one truly did not notice physical characteristics.

The aim of this book is to remind each reader of his uniqueness, his potential, and his importance in life and in the sight of God. We shall look at the beauty of the internal, the external, and the eternal.

To follow the recommendations of this book necessitates a renewed look at our bodies, our habits, our minds, our thoughts, our appearance, our faith.

Plato wrote, around 428-340 B.C., "The life which is unexamined is not worth living." Perhaps we could paraphrase this to say that the life which is unexamined is not all that it could be.

Our bodies are the temple of the Holy Spirit (I Corinthians 6:19). We are the stewards of a magnificent possession — our body, our life, our influences, our potential.

There is nothing on earth more important than a human being. And you are a human being.

But you are more. You are special. You are not just a body; you are somebody.

The greatest challenge in life is to be and to become the very best that one is capable of becoming.

The method is simple. We take what we have and what we are, and day by day, we determine to improve, polish, and perfect all that we are capable of becoming.

Doing this is both a conscious and a subconscious effort. Work, responsibility, illness, problems, and tears must, of necessity, take us away from ourselves. But the goal is to plant that seed of desire and determination, that, regardless of circumstances, will help us to become, with God's help, all that we can be.

There is nothing on earth more wonderful than a beautiful life filled with discipline, concern, and growth toward all that comes from within, all that is seen without, and all that will be — forever.

Will Rogers wrote: "I never met a man I didn't like."[1] Think for a moment. Can you truthfully say that you have ever met a person that you did not think was beautiful, or had the potential for being beautiful, in some way?

Maybe life is not always what we planned or hoped. Austin Dobson wrote: "I intended an ode, and it turned to a sonnet." And life is often like that. We intend one thing, and it turns out another.

As I have written this book, I have been reminded again and again that there is nothing new under the sun and that "I am a part of all that I have met."[2]

Over more than four decades, I have read, thought, remembered, believed, and considered many ideas that I have met. There is no way to trace many seed that have sprouted, produced, shed, produced seed, and grown again. I have given credit wherever I could. It is not my aim to claim any ideas as original. Our thoughts are all a part of the great universe of man. So if you read a line, and you say, "I have heard that before," you are probably correct. You may even find a thought from yourself — for you, too, have become a part of me as we have walked and talked and worked together. Again, there is nothing new under the sun.

I do not claim nor proclaim any startling theories or magnificent wonders, but if you will walk with me through the pages of this book, I believe that your journey will not have been in vain.

Remember what John Keats said:

"A thing of beauty is a joy forever;
    Its loveliness increases; it can never
        Pass into nothingness."

And that applies to the internal, the external, and the eternal.

Chapter 2

You Are Beautiful in Many Ways

One out of four beds in the United States is occupied by mental patients — about 330,000.

Fifteen percent of all Americans are affected by mental disorders every year.

About fifteen percent of the people who visit doctors with physical complaints have emotional problems that are partly or wholly responsible.

Mental illness is America's number one social problem.

In the United States, mental illness costs over thirty-eight billion dollars a year.[1]

Mental illness is often attributed to physical causes, environment, heredity, or other influences.

Yet, I believe there is another factor involved in mental illness. After considering many labels, I decided to call it *human neglect*. I am convinced that many people are mentally ill and are taking sedatives and tranquilizers today because no one ever recognized the unique beauty of that person or praised and encouraged that person's unique, distinct attributes. Thirty thousand Americans commit suicide each year. Suicide is second only to accidents as a cause of death among youths fifteen to twenty. For every suicide, there are ten attempts.

God is beautiful. All that He made is beautiful in its own way. Our duty is to find that beauty in others and to recognize it and to praise it. There is a spark of divinity in every human life: that spark is beautiful.

It could be a beautiful
  smile
    voice
      body
        walk
          movement.

It could be a beautiful
  nose
    complexion
      hair
        legs.

It could be a beautiful attitude
  of compassion
    of caring
      of being there at the right moment.

It could be the ability to express oneself
  in speaking
    in singing
      in writing.

It could be a special talent
  in listening
    in caring
      in touching.

It could be a special accomplishment
  in cooking
    in sewing

```
        in housekeeping
          in letter writing
            in knitting
              in painting.

To do, to be, to see: these three—
   in one
      in some
        in many . . .
          You are beautiful.
```

A popular song a few years ago emphasized the philosophy: "Everything is beautiful in its own way."[2] This truth sets forth two challenges:

1. To find beauty in others and to praise it
2. To cultivate and perfect beauty in our own lives

A famous, anonymous quotation states: "What you are is God's gift to you: what you make of yourself is your gift to God."

Harriet Beecher Stowe wrote: "In all ranks of life, the human heart yearns for the beautiful, and the beautiful things that God makes are His gift to all alike."

How many of us are sane and happy and normal today because someone cared, because someone encouraged us and recognized the good in us? How many of us have felt alone and cast away with the same feeling that David had when he wrote in Psalm 142:4 — ". . . No man cared for my soul."

Fourteen million Americans over the age of thirty use sleeping pills regularly. Does this imply anxiety, fear, unrest? Over 2.5 million people in America suffer from acute depression.[3] Twenty million people in our country suffer from mental illness.[4]

Is there anything we can do? Let us consider the thought of this version of a challenging thought:

"I shall pass through this world but once.
Any good therefore,
That I can do, or any kindness
That I can show to
Any human being, let me do
It now. Let me not defer
Or neglect it, for I shall not
Pass this way again."[5]

Henry Drummond

Chapter 3

Simplicity

This book advocates ultimate simplicity.

Marquis de Vauvenargues advised: "When a thought is too weak to be simply expressed, it is clear proof that it should be rejected."

In WALDEN, Henry David Thoreau wrote: "Our life is frittered away by detail . . . simplify, simplify."

Our minds are filled with too much clutter.

Our wardrobes are filled with too many items.

Socrates, in looking at a mass of things at a sale was reputed to have said: "How many things I have no need of."

Our homes are filled with unnecessary pieces that we must move, dust, and clean.

Our schedules are filled with meetings, appointments, and responsibilities, that, under false assumption, we feel are necessary to our fulfillment.

How many of us have read diets too complicated to follow?

How many of us have tried to read descriptions of exercise routines, only to give up because the instructions were wordy and confusing?

"In character, in manners, in style, in all things, the supreme
excellence is simplicity."

Henry Wadsworth Longfellow

Let's read that one again:

"In character
    in manners
       in style
       in all things
          the supreme excellence
             is simplicity."   Longfellow

Richard Steele stated: "Simplicity, of all things, is
the hardest to be copied." Ralph Waldo Emerson said
that "nothing is more simple than greatness; indeed, to
be simple is to be great." "The greatest truths are the
simplest: and so are the greatest men," wrote John
Hare. And "There is majesty in simplicity," penned
Alexander Pope.

Pope John XXIII (Pope from 1958-1963) wrote: "I
must strip my vines of all useless foliage and concentrate on what is truth, justice, and charity . . . The older
I grow, the more clearly I perceive the dignity and
winning beauty of simplicity in thought, conduct, and
speech . . ."

The ultimate aim of all knowledge is simplification so
that it may become practical wisdom. To be useful,
even the most complicated and profound must be
simplified. Successful living is a constant effort toward
simplification which will lead to victory over the overwhelming and the confusing.

So often, we let clutter and confusion prevent us from
doing the things we should and also from doing them
well.

To simplify life:

Purify the mind through prayer, meditation, quietness, rest, fresh air, sunshine, pure food, fresh water.

Clean your house through packing unnecessary items and giving to the needy unused items.

Clean your house—floors, closets, windows, cabinets—all!

Cleanse and clean all of life—the outer, around and about; the inner soul and spirit, inside and out!

Chapter 4

Counting Good Things

K nowing God is life's greatest blessing — for this is eternal. It is just that simple: it needs no further explanation or emphasis.

Over the years, of all the commencement sermons that I heard, one especially was memorable. The speaker continued to ask, as he enumerated important thoughts of life, "But does God know your name?" This profound question, too, suffices within itself: it needs no exposition.

But what about other good things, other blessing? One night recently, for several hours, I had severe pains in my left foot and leg. Fortunately, aspirin erased the hurt, but during the night, I promised, "When I am free from pain again, I shall never complain about anything again."

I thought of all those who suffer from pain.

For thousands, pain never goes away. Some officials estimate that lower-back pain alone afflicts seven million adults who lose ten to fifteen million work days per year because of pain.

Dr. John J. Bonica, developer of the first pain clinic in this country, at the University of Washington in Seattle, estimates the annual cost of back ailments to be more than seventeen billion dollars including lost work time, hospital bills, and medication.

To be alive is essential, but to be free of pain is, except for God, life's greatest blessing.

> To be free from hunger
> To be free from thirst
> To be warm . . .
> To be able to sleep and rest
> To be able to hope
> To be able to dream . . .
>
> To be able to speak
>   to hear
>   to see
>   to move
>   to write
>   to think . . .
> These are good things.

Never let anybody or anything — houses, lands, money, or anything — rob you of the joy of everyday things that we so often take for granted.

Consider these thoughts from a feature article entitled, "Enjoy What You Have."

> "Do not want what you cannot have. Some
> persons make themselves constantly unhappy
> reaching for what is beyond their grasp
> instead of enjoying what is right at their
> feet. There is far more to be enjoyed from
> a single walk around the block or across a
> field than a whole truckload of chrome-
> plated gadgets.

Enjoy what you have. Appreciate your gifts
and talents, and it will go a long way toward
making you a well-adjusted, efficient, happy
person. To be satisfied or not is a question
only you can answer for yourself. Try it and see."[1]

Author Unknown

We complain, become pessimistic, and even depressed and bitter.

Somewhere, our schools, or Sunday Schools, or families, or community, or maybe even we ourselves, failed us. We failed to learn to count good things, to count blessings.

We are all rich, "filthy rich," as the saying goes.

Many times, I have heard the analysis of wealth illustrated in this way. Suppose someone asked you to sell your hands, your eyes, your ears, your family, your child, your mind. What price would you ask for each? We are rich, very rich.

One who has learned to count blessings is beautiful, for an awareness of God's intangible and tangible gifts to each of us gives serenity and peace that glows and shows in the face. We need to become better stewards of what we have, not strugglers in the massive world of confusion and competition.

"The best things are nearest: breath
in your nostrils, light in your eyes,
flowers at your feet, duties at your
hand, the path of Right just before you.
Then do not grasp at the stars, but do
life's plain, common work as it comes,
certain that daily duties and daily bread
are the sweetest things in life."

Robert Louis Stevenson

"And though I come not within sight of the

castle of my dreams, teach me still to be
thankful for life, and for time's olden
memories that are good and sweet."

Author Unknown

A Louis Harris survey gave the following information concerning what Americans assess to be important. Three personal things stand out: family life, health, and peace of mind. Nationwide, 1,442 adults were included in the survey.

1. 92 percent said that family life is important.
   67 percent said that they are satisfied with family life.
2. 97 percent said that good health is very important.
   54 percent said that they are satisfied.
3. 76 percent felt that having the respect of others is important.
   60 percent are satisfied.
4. 71 percent felt that friends are important.
   64 percent felt that they have such friends.
5. 91 percent felt that peace of mind is very important.
   52 percent are satisfied.
6. 60 percent maintained that work is important:
   43 percent are satisfied.
7. 69 percent felt that education is important.
   25 percent are satisfied with the education they received.
8. 47 percent felt that money is very important.
   25 percent are satisfied with their income.[2]

These ideas indicate that in the 1970's, non-material values were dominant to Americans. Again, family, health, and peace of mind are great, good things — blessings.

Chapter 5

A Positive Self-Image

One of the most overwhelming thoughts is that we have only one first chance of only a few seconds to make a lasting, lifetime impression, as the John Robert Powers School teaches.

I emphasize: our ultimate aim in life is not to make impressions.

But we do.

And again, we do this during the first few seconds when we meet someone for the first time.

Is this frightening?

It need not be.

How can we prepare ourselves for this possible day-by-day experience?

First, we learn to feel comfortable about ourselves. It has something to do with that idea referred to as "a positive self-image."

What is a positive self-image? It is realizing that one is created in the image of God (Genesis 1:27) and that your life, like every other life, is sacred and important.

A positive self-image involves self-respect, acceptance of one's shortcomings, reasonable adjustment to life's disappointments, frustrations and fears, and a command of life that brings freedom from anger, jealousy, covetousness, and hatred.

Second, a positive self-image involves a deep, genuine, sincere feeling about others and one's relationship to other human beings. This involves respect, trust, compassion, caring, love . . .

When we meet another person for the first time, something about our being must say, "I like you. I accept you. Your life is sacred and important, for you are a product of the sacred and for eternity. I may not be able to help you, but I shall do you no harm. I may never see you again, but for this moment, I shall love you and accept you for all the wonder and beauty that you are . . ."

Third, a positive self-image involves poise — quietness, simplicity, sincerity, genuineness. Do not seek to impress, overwhelm, or overshadow.

Fourth, a positive self-image involves a smile — a genuine, spontaneous, natural, love-motivated smile. There is nothing more unattractive or more obvious (or maybe obnoxious is a better word) than an artificial smile that is "acted" to impress. A smile must come from the heart, from the soul. It must come from years of motivation, of concern, feeling, caring, thinking, listening, learning, loving . . .

Fifth, a positive self-image involves self-confidence motivated by cleanliness of body and mind and good grooming, both of body and dress.

So, with a proper attitude about ourselves and others, we go forth to face the inevitable — meeting new people and associating with those we have known.

Let us pause here. Often, eventually, we ask, or are asked, "What is your profession?" Our answers vary: housewife, teacher, doctor, secretary, clerk, lawyer, pharmacist, seamstress, or one of hundreds of others.

But subconsciously, we ought always to recall, not aloud, but silently, "My profession is being a person."

Then, with respect for ourselves and love for mankind, we are ready to go forth to meet the world.

Then what do we do?

We do all that we can to put that person at ease, to make that person feel important, to make that person feel comfortable and at ease with us.

How do we do this?

After we say, "How do you do?" or "I'm so happy to meet you," we try to find a simple, sincere question to ask or a statement to make to encourage the person to talk about himself, or to talk about anything that interests him or her. What we sometimes refer to as "small talk" or trite conversation will promote and perpetuate a lasting friendship that will lead to deeper thoughts and deeper relationships.

Ask simple questions or make statements that motivate responses.

1. Are you weary of travel?
2. That is a handsome briefcase or ring or pendant.
3. What is your hometown?
4. I know someone from your hometown. She is Jayne Smithers.
5. Tell me about your product.
6. Isn't this a lovely party?
7. You look handsome in that suit, lovely in that dress.

Once the person begins to talk about himself, become

a good listener — and listen, listen, listen. But listening is another chapter.

If the person asks about you, answer quickly, simply, briefly, and sincerely. Then, immediately, ask another question or make another statement that turns the person's thoughts to himself.

By doing this, you will make a good first impression.

If you are sincere, you will have added one more moment in your life as a charming, friendly person.

> "This above all: to thine own self be
>   true,
> And it must follow, as the night the
>   day,
> Thou canst not then be false to any
>   man."
>   William Shakespeare
>   HAMLET, Act I, Scene III, Line 75

This involves loyalty and allegiance — to one's self and to others.

Chapter 6

Praise

O ne of the most powerful, profound truths that I have ever read is by an unknown writer who said, "Anything scarce is valuable: praise, for example."

Again,

> "Anything scarce is valuable,
>   Praise, for example."

Napoleon wrote: "An army's effectiveness depends on its size, training, experience, and morale . . . and morale is worth more than all the other factors combined."

Praise must be simple, short, and sincere. It must be honest recognition of those endearing, worthy qualities in others, whether they be physical, spiritual, emotional, mental, or others.

Seeing beauty in others and recognizing attributes must not be motivated as the mother who bathed and dressed her young son and said, "Now, you're sweeter and better than the other grandchildren because you're clean and 'dressed up.' "

The young child stood on the front porch and said to the other children, "Hey, look! I'm better than you are because I'm cleaner than you."

Our life touches dozens of lives each day. Many of these people help us in special ways. Use as many opportunities as possible to say:

> I love you.
> I'm proud of you.
> I appreciate you.
> I admire you and all you do.
> I respect you and all that you are.

John Ruskin once said that failing to praise a person could lead to two things: the chance of driving him from the right way for lack of encouragement, and the certainty of depriving ourselves of one of the very happiest privileges in life . . .

Praise is included in the "Ten Commandments for Living with People," by an unknown writer:

1. Speak to people. Nothing is so nice as a cheerful greeting.
2. Smile at people. It takes seventy-two muscles to frown, fourteen to smile.
3. Call people by name. The sweetest sound is one's own name.
4. Be friendly and helpful. If you want friends, be a friend.
5. Be cordial. Speak and act in such a way as to demonstrate that everything you do is a genuine pleasure.
6. Be genuinely interested in people. Just try and you can like almost everyone.
7. Be generous with praise. And be courteous with criticism.
8. Be considerate of others. There are often three sides to a controversy: yours, his, and the right side.
9. Be alert to give help. What we do for others' lives is immortal.

10. Add to all this a sense of humor, loads of patience, and a dash of humility, and you will be rewarded manyfold.

Chapter 7

Adjusting to Others

Regardless of religious beliefs, scientific knowledge, or medical journals, common sense and everyday observations help us to understand that most human lives move in days of strength and weakness and depression and happiness. Regardless of faith or philosophy, human attitudes and feelings change; and emotions and reactions are affected.

Being beautiful means accepting others' moods — the good days and the bad, the up's and down's of physical and emotional strength.

The ability to get along with people affects personal happiness and success in all phases of life.

This adjusting to one's family, friends, and co-workers must be genuine on our part so that it will not cause us unnecessary stress. It must also be accepted and understood as genuine by others who observe our adjustment to, and acceptance of, them. There is no attribute less becoming than shallowness and superficiality, which this book talks about elsewhere. Never, not even to one soul, must we appear compassionate and understanding, and then judge, condemn, or criticize when one's back is turned.

In dealing with the emotions of others, these ideas may help:

1. Laura Archera Huxley's book title, YOU ARE NOT THE TARGET,[1] says it all. Often, almost always, when people are snappy, ill, unkind, inconsiderate, or negative toward us, we are not the target. It is as simple as that. Allow people to vent their anger. Let them scream, snap, and yell. Listen. Wait. If you will wait a few minutes, you, in quietness and peace, can determine whether you are really the target.

2. Biorhythms, or the biorhythm theory, contend that there are three rhythmic cycles that determine, or affect drastically, human actions: the physical cycle of 23 days; the emotional, 28 days; and the intellectual, 33 days.

Each cycle has a critical period for about 24 hours when nothing seems to go right. According to the biorhythm theory, all one has to do is to count onward from his or her birth date to determine error-prone days on the twenty-third day, the twenty-eighth, and the thirty-third, counting each from birth, of course. Generally, these must be figured by experts or computers.

Another version of the biorhythm theory is that the first half of each cycle is positive and the second is negative. The day when one switches from the positive to the negative — or back again — is termed a "critical" day. If two cycles experience a switch at the same time, this is a double critical day. If all three cycles are changing the same day, it is a triple day. It is thought that triple critical days occur about once every seven years.

Whether we accept the biorhythm theory, it is only a common sense reaction-adjustment that we be more aware of our emotions and our actions at critical times when we do not seem to be at our best.

Another theory is the effect of the full moon. Policemen and firemen report more activity during the full moon. Psychiatric ward attendants report more erratic, disturbed behavior during the full moon period.

Again, whether we accept the biorhythmic theory, or the full moon observations, or any other theory, is not the point. The idea is that we must recognize the varying moods of people and adjust to them.

Hunger, stress, fatigue, psychological and physiological factors, as well as environmental and generic factors, affect us and make us the person that we are. Again, many negative feelings, fears, and frustrations come to us because we are tired, hungry, or ill.

Anyone who has ever been a part of a family, attended public school, or held a public job does not have to be told that human moods and emotions, as well as physical strength and intellectual ability, vary, for most people, day by day. None of us are really "always and forever the same."

Consideration of the possibility of days of strength and weakness may be a key factor in understanding moods.

Perhaps Mary Carolyn Davies best expressed our adjustment to others when she wrote: "If I had known what trouble you were bearing . . . What griefs were in the silence of your face . . . I would have been more gentle and more caring . . . And tried to give you gladness for a space . . . I would have brought more warmth into the place . . . If I had known . . . ."

Chapter 8

Love and the Family

In marriage and in the family, love, or the lack of it, shows in the face, in the voice, in the eyes, in the step, in all that one is.

The following poem, framed and displayed in my parents' bedroom for over fifty years, perhaps expresses the essence of a happy marriage. Remember, this book is an effort in simplicity and serenity.

Companionship

It isn't that we talk so much:
   Sometimes the evening through,
You do not say a word to me,
   I do not talk to you.
I sit beside the reading lamp,
   You like your easy chair,
And it is joy enough to me
   To know that you are there.

It isn't that we go so much:
   Sometimes we like to roam,
To concert or to theater,
   But best of all is home.
Our lives are fitted each to each,

In all our likes we share,
And it is joy enough to me
To know that you are there.

It isn't that you tell to me
The things I've come to know;
For some things are too deep for words
And love is surely so.
You only have to touch my hand
To learn how much I care,
And it is joy enough for me
To know that you are there.

By Anne Campbell

Charlie Shedd wrote: "Marriage is not finding the right person, but being the right person."

This quotation by an unknown writer says much:

Woman
    was created from the rib of man.
She was not made
    from his head
        to top him
    nor from his feet
        to be trampled on.

She was made
    from his side
        to be equal to him
    from under his arm
        to be protected by him:
    from near his heart
        to be loved by him.

These thoughts from Ann Landers:

Love

"Love is friendship that has caught fire. It is quiet understanding, mutual confidence, sharing, and forgiving. It is loyalty through good and bad. It settles for less than perfection and makes allowances for human weaknesses.

"Love is content with the present, its hopes for the future, and it doesn't brood over the past. It's the day-in-day-out chronicle of irritations, problems, compromises, small disappointments, big victories, and working toward common goals.

"If you have love in your life, it can make up for a great many things that you lack. If you don't have it, no matter what else there is, it is not enough."[1]

I like what Herbert Hoover said about children: "A boy has two jobs: one is just being a boy. The other is growing to be a man." The same is true of a girl — just being a girl and growing to be a woman. What jobs these are!

Below is a favorite, clipped many years ago:

To My Son

I will not say to you, "This is the Way; walk in it."
For I do not know your way or where the Spirit may call you.
It may be to paths I have never trod or ships on the sea leading
    to unimagined lands afar,
Or haply, to a star!
Or yet again
Through dark and perilous places racked with pain and full of
    fear
Your road may lead you far away from me or near . . .
I cannot guess or guide, but only stand aside.
Just this I say:
I know for every truth there is a way for each to walk, a right
    for each to choose, a truth to use.
And though you wander far, your soul will know the true path
    when you find it.
Therefore, go!
I will fear nothing for you day or night!
I will not grieve at all because your light is called by some new
    name:

Truth is the same!
It matters nothing to call it star or sun . . .
All light is one.

Author Unknown

And another favorite from Ann Landers:

Hold Fast the Summer
It is the beauty of the day
and all of it contains
   The laughter and the work
and finally the sleep. The
quiet.
   Oh, September, do not
put your weight upon my
mind.
   For I know he will be
going.
   This son of mine who is
now a man—he must go.
   Time will lace my thoughts
with joyous years
   The walls will echo his
"Hello." His caring will be
around each corner.
   His tears will be tucked
into our memory book.
   Life calls him beyond our
reach—to different walls,
   New faces, shiny halls,
shy smiles, many places.
   Greater learning—he must
go. But wait, before he
leaves.
   Be sure he knows you
love him. Hide the lump in
your throat as you hug him.
   He'll soon be home again—
but he will be different.

The little boy will have
disappeared.
    How I wish I could take
September and shake it.
    For it came too soon.
    I must look to the beauty
of each new day
    And silently give thanks.[2]
                    Author Unknown

Life is brief, at longest. I think of family and friends as
Henry Wadsworth Longfellow wrote:

"Ships that pass in the night and speak
    to each other in passing; only a signal
    shown and a distant voice in the darkness.
  So in the ocean of life, we pass and look and
    speak to one another, and a voice, then
    darkness again and silence."

Or consider the beauty and the truth in William
Henry Harrison's thoughts:

Ah, friends, dear friends,
As the years go on and heads get gray,
How fast the guests do go.
Touch hands, tough hands with those who stay:
Strong hands to weak, old hands to young.
Around the Christmas board, touch hands.
The false forget, the foe forgive:
For every guest will go and every fire burn low—
and empty cabin stand.
Forget, forgive. For who may say that Christmas Day may
ever come to host or guest again . . .
Touch hands.

The following poem is often reprinted with the author unknown. The version below is attributed by one source to Roy Croft.

I Love You

I love you,
Not only for what you are
But what I am
When I am with you.

I love you,
Not only for what
You have made of yourself,
But for what
You are making of me.

I love you for
For the part of me
That you bring out;
I love you
For putting your hand
Into my heaped-up heart
And passing over
All the foolish, weak things
That you can't help
Dimly seeing there.
And for drawing out
Into the light
All the beautiful longings
That no one else had looked
Quite far enough to find.

I love you because you
Are helping to make
Of the lumber of my life
Not a tavern, but a temple.
Out of the works
Of my everyday life
Not a reproach, but a song.

I love you
Because you have done
More than any creed
Could have done,
And more than any fate
Could have done
To make me happy.

You have done it
Without a touch
Without a word
Without a sign.
You have done it
By being yourself.
Perhaps that is what
Being a friend means,
After all.[3]

Roy Croft

Chapter 9

Putting Sparkle in Your Eyes

If you want to put sparkle in your eyes, try love.

Look at the young bride-to-be. Look at a child's eyes at Christmas. Look at the glow of an expectant mother.

My mother came to help me arrange a new middle school library. She was already tired from summer's work — canning, freezing, homemaking, and farm work. Our work in the new school was time-consuming and fatiguing. But after a few days, there was a new glow in her face, a renewed sparkle in her eyes. She was working hard, but she was working with meaning — and love.

Let us look at what some of the masters have said:

> "The greatest happiness of life is the
> conviction that we are loved, loved for
> ourselves, or rather, in spite of ourselves."
> Victor Hugo

> "In making others happy, you will be happy,
> too. For the happiness you give away,
> returns to shine on you."
> Helen Steiner Rice

"The best portion of a good man's life
is the little nameless, unremembered
acts of love."

William Wordsworth

"Where there is faith, there is love,
Where there is love, there is peace,
Where there is peace, there is God,
Where there is God, there is no need."

Leo Tolstoy

"I am only one
But still I am one.
I cannot do everything
But still I can do something
And because I cannot do everything,
I will not refuse to do the something that I can do."

Edward Everett Hale

"It is good that men should think,
but it is indispensable that men
should love."

Bernard Bell

"At one time, through love, all
things come together into one.
At another time, through strife's
hatred, they are borne each of
them apart."

Empedocles, FRAGMENT 17

"I have held many things in my
hands, and I have lost them all,
but whatever I have placed in
God's hands, that I still possess."

Martin Luther

"Do all the good you can,
By all the means you can,
In all the ways you can,
In all the places you can,

At all the times you can,
To all the people you can,
As long as ever you can.

John Wesley

"When you are crossing the desert,
plant trees — for you may be coming
back the same way in your old age,
when you will be glad of the shade."

A Persian Proverb

"The actions of men are like the index
of a book: they point out what is
most remarkable in them."

Heinrich Heine (1791-1856)

"No one could tell where my soul might be;
I searched for God, and He eluded me:
I sought my brother out, and found all three."

Ernest Crosby

"Good actions ennoble us, and we are the
sons of our own deeds."

Cervantes

Say It Now

If you have a friend worth loving,
Love him. Yes, and let him know
That you love him, ere life's evening
Tinge his brow with sunset glow . . .

If you hear a song that thrills you
Sung by any child of song,
Praise it. Do not let the singer
Wait deserved praises long . . .

If you hear a prayer that moves you
By its humble, pleading tone,
Join it. Do not let the seeker
Bow before his God alone . . .

If your work is made more easy
By a friendly, helping hand,
Say so. Speak out brave and truly
Ere the darkness veil the land . . .
Author Unknown

Love

There is no difficulty that love will not conquer
no disease that enough love will not heal
no door that enough love will not open
no gulf that enough love will not bridge
no wall that enough love will not throw down
no sin that enough love will not redeem.

It makes no difference
how deeply seated may be the trouble
how hopeless the outlook
how muddled the tangle
how great the mistake
A sufficient amount of love
will dissolve it all.
If only you could love enough
you would be
the happiest
and most powerful being
in the world.
Emmet Fox

Prayer of Saint Francis

Lord, make me an instrument of Thy Peace.
Where there is hatred, let me sow Love;
Where there is injury, Pardon;
Where there is doubt, Faith;
Where there is despair, Hope;
Where there is darkness, Light, and
Where there is sadness, Joy.

O Divine Master,
Grant that I may not so much

Seek to be consoled as to Console;
To be understood as to Understand;
To be loved, as to Love;
For it is in Giving that we receive;
It is in Pardoning that we are pardoned;
And it is in Dying that we are born to Eternal Life.
                                    Saint Francis of Assisi

During the Great Depression of the 1930's, a neighbor's child died a few hours after birth. Daddy and the other neighbors gathered beneath the trees in our yard to build a small, wood casket. Mama lined it with baby blankets.

While the casket was being built, someone suggested that the neighbors try to collect food or clothing or money for the family that had lost the child. Although it seems incredible today, almost no one had anything. Money, especially, was scarce.

An old man who had joined the small group expressed an unforgettable thought. He spoke of a family that had enough to share if its members had chosen to do so. He said, "No need to go to that family, They have never given anybody anything, and they never will. They keep it all for themselves . . ."

Dr. Albert Schweitzer, medical missionary, built his philosophy and life's work around the idea of service. In 1952, he received the Nobel Prize for Peace for his life of service to others. Among many other things, he established a hospital in French Equatorial Africa. Later, he used the $33,000 Nobel Prize money to expand the hospital and to establish a leper colony.

Dr. Schweitzer spoke many beautiful thoughts, but I like this one especially:

"You know what I would really like to do if I had time? Just once or twice, to get up without feeling tired and to go to bed without knowing how many things are still left undone. What a luxury that would be!"[1]

Do not deny yourself the greatest joy on earth: service to others through love.

Do not deny yourself the greatest aid to human beauty: sparkle in your eyes from service to others through love.

It's in Your Face

You don't have to tell how you live each day
You don't have to say if you work or play,
A tried, true barometer serves in its place,
However you live will show in your face.

The false, the deceit that you bear in your heart
Will not stay inside where it first got a start,
For sinew and blood are a thin veil of lace,
What you wear in your heart you wear in your face.

Author Unknown

Chapter 10

The Art of Listening

As a young college student, I was asked to attend a conference on listening. Puzzled initially, I was to learn later, in depth, that listening is an art, a skill, comparable to reading, writing, thinking, speaking, and reasoning.

During the conference I realized that I was often a poor listener.

Hearing is done with the ears. Listening is done with the mind as well as the ears, and we might add, often with the heart.

How many times did we say as a child, "Mama, you're not listening to me!" Or how many times has our mother or dad or a teacher or a friend asked, "Hey, are you listening to me?"

Listen to learn. Listen to succeed. Listen to improve relationships. Listen to care. Listen to help.

Be careful about listening to advise. It is perhaps better to repeat a person's care and say, "What do you really want to do?"

Listen with eye contact, with facial expressions. One

of the most frustrating experiences is to talk to someone and have that person look away. Do not think about what you are going to say next. Concentrate on what the person is saying. Listen, really listen. Use simple gestures such as a nod of the head, or a simple movement of the body, to show that you are following.

Psychologists tell us that if we listen, really listen, we can recall more than fifty percent of the information we hear. Someone has said: "Good listeners are popular people because every person has a need to be heard."

Often, over the years, when I was tired or weary or troubled, I would have the uncontrollable yearning to go home. Often, Daddy or Mama would say as we talked, "Joyce, don't you want something to eat or drink . . . Would you like some potatoes to take home or some apples or some pickles?"

And in quiet desperation I would say, "No, I just want us to talk." What I really meant was, "I just want you to listen to me."

According to Dr. Leo Hawkins, human development specialist with the North Carolina Agricultural Extension Service, North Carolina State University, Raleigh, "Listening Is One of the Nicest Things to Do for Children."

He provides these guidelines to better communication between parents and children as well as between adults:

> "Be interested and show it. Genuine concern and a lively curiosity encourage others to speak freely. Interest also sharpens your attention and builds on itself.

> "Tune in to the other person. Try to understand his or her needs, viewpoint, assumptions, and system of beliefs.

> "Hold your fire. Avoid jumping to conclusions and hear the

speaker out. Plan your response only after you are certain that you have gotten the whole message.

"Look for the main ideas. Avoid being distracted by details and focus on the key issue. You may have to dig hard to find it.

"Watch for feelings. Often people talk to "get something off their chest." Feelings, not facts, may be the main issue.

"Monitor your own feelings and point of view. Each of us listens differently. Our convictions and emotions filter and even distort what we hear. Be aware of your own attitudes, prejudices, cherished beliefs, and your emotional reaction to the message.

"Notice nonverbal language. A shrug, a smile, a nervous laugh, gestures, facial expressions, and body positions speak volumes. Learn to read them.

"Give the other person the benefit of the doubt. We often enter conversations with our minds already made up, at least partially, on the basis of past experience. Pre-judgments can shut out new messages.

"Work at listening. Hearing is passive. Our nervous system does the work. Listening is active: it takes mental effort and attention.

"Get feedback. Make certain you are really listening. Ask a question and confirm with the speaker what he or she actually said."[1]

You are beautiful when you learn to listen.

Chapter 11

Concerning Men

Sometimes society is unfair. It takes something away from us without giving us anything in return, not even a substitute.

Such is the case when society says that we cannot say that men are beautiful.

Society demands and commands that we say that one is handsome, exciting, good looking, or nice looking, but even then, we are moving into the realm beyond physical attractiveness as related to looks or appearance. We can say that a woman is pretty, lovely, beautiful, charming, elegant, attractive, graceful, radiant, and gorgeous, but no such words, nor synonyms for these words, are available to describe the physical appearance or attributes of a man.

Women talk much about women's liberation and women's rights. But deep inside, we realize that in God's divine plan, he included men to make the world complete. They are as essential as the air, the rain, the sky, the food we eat. They make the circle complete. They are the link in the unbroken chain — or the chain that breaks.

Remember when Daddy's strong hand checked your forehead
during a fever, and the fever almost went away.

Remember when he picked you up in his strong arms the day you broke your arm and the pain almost left you.

Remember that day that a doctor's strong, calm voice said that you needed surgery, but assured you that everything would be all right.

Remember those trips to the dentist when you were scared to death and the dentist sat down beside you, spoke gently and said, "This will hurt a little, maybe a minute, but not for long . . ."

Remember that morning strong arms lifted you gently onto the stretcher of the ambulance, and you suddenly felt that you would survive in spite of the pain and fear.

Remember that time your car stalled just after sunset, and you were all alone on that deserted road. He came along and said, "Let me check to see whether a belt or bolt is loose."

Remember that flat tire? How many women can change a flat tire?

Remember when you had gone the last mile of the way and he said, "Don't worry. I'll take care of everything."

What does one say to a man, even in "extreme circumstances such as love," to express admiration, respect, or to compliment physique?

We break the rule. We reach forth with a firm, heart-motivated handshake of feeling and respect, and we say to one who really deserves it: "You are wonderful: you really are! And you are indeed a beautiful person." Ask any man whether he would be offended by these words.

Whisper to the one you love in that quiet moment: "Golly, you're wonderful — and a beautiful human being." Ask him later whether he was offended. You don't dare! You already know the answer!

Chapter 12

No More Trophies

Among other things, we are a trophy-award-reward oriented society. We give (luckily) and expect (unluckily) praise and prestige.

As children, we behave well and we are rewarded with candy. We go to school and we are rewarded if we get a good report card. In high school we become cheerleaders and marshals and presidents, and we get medals and ribbons and pats-on-the-back. We send home grade sheets and Mama and Daddy are proud.

We finish college with high honors — or at least, with a diploma. The world looks at us and calls us educated, whether we are or not — and we walk a little taller. We get married and we are queen for a day. We buy or build a new home and we move in with joy. We get a public job, and we are inspired by the newness of the new work and the new paycheck. Then comes the new baby, and we are again queen of the world — or at least, queen of the family, especially the grandparents. Everything is on the up and up, for a long time, even for several years.

Then suddenly, about midway, there are no more

trophies. No more grades sent home, no more medals received, no more children in the nest. Life is half gone, and we feel useless, unimportant, and unneeded. What then?

I was saying all this at Atlantic Christian College, Wilson, North Carolina. I paused. During the pause, a young coed, thinking that my story had ended, that one day there would be no more trophies, questioned: "My goodness, what next? What do we do when we reach this stage?"

"That's the heart of the matter," I said. "You don't receive trophies, but you can give them in a million ways."

"Oh, I see," she said, sounding relieved. "You are right."

Isn't it beautiful that life is divided about half way so that we both receive and give? There is an overlapping of giving and receiving throughout life, of course, but so often, days are divided so that there comes a time of "no more trophies."

How does one give trophies?

The answer is obvious. Constantly, we look and listen for ways to help others, directly or indirectly.

What does this have to do with beauty?

Again, the answer is obvious. It has something to do with that special sparkle of happiness in knowing that life extends far beyond ourselves — and far beyond . . .

Chapter 13

Joy in Patriotism

When you are driving to work and someone is hoisting the flag, do you have an uncontrollable urge to stop to watch?

When "The Star Spangled Banner" is played and sung before a game, do you choke a bit before it is finished?

Can you sing "My country 'tis of thee, sweet land of liberty" without getting that indescribable feeling of a prayer?

Al Capp wrote: "We have taught our children to demand American comforts, American privileges, to demand everything from America to make their lives easier. But we haven't taught them to love America."

When I was a child, in the general assembly of our Sunday School, my dad was often asked to pray. Always, before he ended the prayer, he prayed for our country and its leaders and thanked God for our land of freedom and opportunity. Doing this became a trademark, an expected thing. Even though it may have been repetitive, I doubt that any young person who grew up in that Sunday School has forgotten that concern for our nation and our homeland.

During my youth, while I was in grades one through eight, all students in our school at Saratoga, North Carolina, under the principalship of such men as W. J. Barefoot and J. A. Williams, and others, assembled in the auditorium for devotions, the pledge of allegiance, announcements, and group singing. Always, daily, we sang "America," "The Star Spangled Banner," and often "The Battle Hymn of the Republic," "Columbia, the Gem of the Ocean," and "God Bless America." During the years of World War II, we sang all the patriotic songs that were so popular — dozens of them. Except for church songs, these were basically the songs of our lives, and we hummed them and sang them, consciously and spontaneously, day and night.

When the hostages came home from Iran in the early days of January, 1981, I thought over and over of the poem we had learned in school, and then one morning, in assembly at our middle school, in thanksgiving for the hostages' return, I used these famous words by Henry Van Dyke:

"So it's home again, and home again, America for me!
My heart is turning home again, and there I long to be,
In the land of youth and freedom, beyond the ocean bars,
Where the air is full of sunlight and the flag is full of stars."

As I grew up, everything that I read or saw inspired love of country. Years later, on the occasion of America's Bicentennial, I penned these words, gleaned from thoughts I had read, sung, or heard — or which I had found in my heart.

Bicentennial Prayer

Our Father,

Under Thy Divine guidance and knowledge, two hundred years ago, "our forefathers brought forth on this continent a new nation, conceived in liberty and dedicated to the proposition that all men are created equal."

In the beauty and quietness of this moment, we lift our hearts in gratitude for our America — our great land of freedom and opportunity, where "government of the people, by the people, and for the people" has not perished from the face of the earth.

We thank you for our land — for its "spacious skies, its amber waves of grain, its purple mountain majesties, above the fruited plain."

For its fertile fields, waterfalls, rivers and quiet streams — its bounty that feeds our people and those of other great nations.

We thank Thee for our people — the men who wrote the Declaration of Independence, the Constitution, the Pledge of Allegiance, the American's Creed, and our laws . . .

For those who braved the storms of Plymouth Rock, stood as Minutemen at Concord, and lay in rags on frozen earth at Valley Forge — for the sacrifice of life and limb at Gettysburg, the Argonne Forest, in Normandy, the Philippines, Korea and Vietnam . . .

For those who conquered the tiny polio germ or took us to the farthest corners of the moon . . .

For fishermen, farmers, miners, truck drivers, teachers, ministers, housewives, policemen, lawyers and countless others of the great masses who were born here and who have come from the ends of the earth —

who work with heart and hands to make this nation good and great.

We thank Thee for our young people to whom we pass the blessing of preserving our great heritage to all posterity.

We thank Thee for our land and for our people, but most of all, for the hearts of men . . .

Men who know the importance of honor, truth and courage who wrote "We the people" and "We hold these truths to be self-evident" . . .

Men of justice, faith, peace and brotherhood, for we know that "though we speak with the tongues of men and angels and have not love, we are as sounding brass and a tinkling cymbal."

May this hour that has brought us together, and the occasion of our America's Bicentennial bind the wounds of prejudice, unrest, uncertainty, and discontent, and raise us to higher, nobler strengths in Thee.

So that Old Glory may still wave "in the dawn's early light," and our land may still "be bright with freedom's holy light" . . .

"Forgive us our debts" to Thee and to others . . .

Forgive our indifference and ingratitude.

Grant unto us "hands that rock the cradle," men who lead onward and upward, and a Maker who loves us . . .

And with this we humbly ask that Thou wilt "give us men," real men — for "a time like this demands strong minds, great hearts, true faith, and ready hands"

for our America

for one another

and for Thee. Amen

(Written for use at the ceremony designating Wilson County a Bicentennial Community)

Consider the ideas in this essay which I also wrote during the Bicentennial year.

Taxes Are the Rent I Pay

Taxes are the rent that I pay to live in America.

Taxes are the price I pay for freedom—freedom to move about freely, day or night, to go where I want to go, work where I want to work, buy what I want to buy, play where I want to play, rest where I want to rest — freedom to live, to love, to laugh, to pray; to run, to scream, to rejoice, and to labor — and to lie down at night without fear of a knock on the door by a soldier who says, "Come with me."

Taxes are the price I pay for the highway patrol, the fireman, the policeman, and the mail carrier.

Taxes are the price I pay for the salaries of men who help make the laws of our land.

Taxes are my small portion of the pay received by men who defend our country, day and night — and the men who fought on foreign soil that I might remain safe and free in my homeland.

Taxes are my small part of the fund that went to the family of the soldier who came home in a flag-draped coffin.

Taxes are my small donation to the salaries of men and women who seek a cure for cancer, mental illness, heart disease, and countless other illnesses.

Taxes are my small contribution to the world of hungry, starving children and adults who look to America for relief.

Taxes are my meager portion in the war against aggression, aggression that promises only suppression and enslavement of men's lives and minds.

Taxes are my bit of assistance with education, roads, ecology, and housing.

What is it worth to live in America? How many of us could ever work long enough or hard enough to pay our daily debts for all she has given and still provides?

I scream as loud as the next citizen when my first check for teaching arrives in the fall — and almost one-fourth of it has gone for taxes — State and Federal. But then, when the initial shock is over, I am humbled and ashamed. Again, what is it worth to live in America? What is the price of freedom?

> Give us, O Land, a bit of income for food and raiment, and a place to lay our head when labor is done. But give us, too, enough to share with our homeland, the place of our birth, our heritage of freedom where the joy of work, love, and faith reign supreme.
>
> Author Unknown

In the great classic, SILAS MARNER, George Eliot wrote: "There's debts we can't pay like (we do) money debts . . ." How true! Especially of America! I owe her a debt I can never pay, but taxes are my opportunity to say "Thank you, America, for letting me live in the greatest nation in the world and finally to be buried in the soil of the land I love."

Chapter 14

Solving Problems: Over 40 Ways to Consider

Our problems often come from being unable to solve our problems. Yes, that is what I said: "Many of our problems come from the problems which we cannot seem to solve."

A lovely friend wrote: "Joyce, write something in your new book about how to deal with problems and still be me . . . Write something practical and realistic, not unrealistic . . . Tell us how to solve problems and to use the solutions to realize more fully one's ideal self . . ."

After I read her request, my first thought was: "My goodness. I cannot solve my own problems. That is my main problem — not being able to solve my problems."

Yet, each of us, in her or his own way, for good physical and mental health, must find solutions to everyday problems.

Reactions to life, problem solving, run in cycles of change, as does fashion. Many of us have witnessed "the me generation," "letting it all hang out," "doing one's own thing," and "suppression of nothing, expression of all.'' These ideas may work for some, but eventually, we return basically, to a different method. Perhaps there are not so many dangerous results from patience, perseverance, serenity, self-control, and thought as one sometimes thinks.

Whenever appropriate or needed, consider these in analyzing problems and seeking solutions to them:

1. Wait three days.

    A really old black friend recommended this idea. She said, ''As Christ was in the earth three days, so I let my problems rest with God for three days. Then, if I must do something, I do it.''

2. Say over and over, ''Even this shall pass away.''

    Consider these lines from ''Even This Shall Pass Away,'' by Theodore Tilton:

    > ''Once in Persia reigned a king
    > Who upon his signet ring
    > Graved a maxim true and wise,
    > Which if held before the eyes,
    > Gave his counsel at a glance
    > Fit for every change and chance.
    > Solemn words, and these are they:
    > 'Even this shall pass away.' ''

3. Be honest with yourself.

    Do not fool or deceive yourself about love, work, debts, diets, or problems — about anything. Nancy Lammeter said in George Eliot's SILAS MARNER: ''Nothing is ever as good as it seems beforehand—nothing.''

    Say again and again with the sage, ''I have to live with myself, so I want myself to be fit to know.'' Ask yourself, ''Can I live with my actions or reactions? Which will be worse, this, or my reactions to my actions?''

4. Do not jump to conclusions.

Give things time. Pericles wrote: ''Wait for the wisest of all counselors—Time.'' Plutarch said: ''Perseverance is more prevailing than violence; and many things which cannot be overcome when they are together yield themselves up when taken little by little.''

5. Pass from out of the midst of those to whom you are allergic.

We are physical beings, not spiritual beings. We are mortals, not yet immortals. In our human way, we react to people, favorably or unfavorably. Some people just naturally ''rub us wrong,'' or ''get on our nerves.'' Often we hear someone say, ''I can't stand so and so . . .''

What does one do? One passes from the midst of the person whenever possible. This does not mean that one despises or dislikes a person. This simply means that one refrains from putting oneself in the presence of a person. After all, there are over two hundred and twenty-five million people in America to love. We cannot associate with everyone personally. Why not let a person that we cannot understand be one of those persons that we eliminate?

What did Jesus do when he was faced with this problem?

> ''And he said, Verily, I say unto you, No prophet is accepted in his own country.
> And all they in the synagogue, when they heard these things, were filled with wrath,

And rose up, and thrust him out of the city, and led him
unto the brow of the hill whereon their city was built,
and they might cast him down headlong.
But he, passing through the midst of them went his way.
And came down to Capernaum, a city of Galilee, and
taught them on the sabbath days.
And they were astonished at his doctrine: for his word
was with power."

From THE HOLY BIBLE
Authorized King James Version
Luke 4:24; 28-32.

Jesus passed from the midst of His enemies and went on to love and work elsewhere. Can we afford to do less? Search for Scriptural passages which tell that the Apostle Paul did the same thing. Read Matthew 10:14 for a synonymous idea. "Shaking the dust from one's feet" is the same as "passing from the midst."

6. Do not think about it (the problem).

One day, in talking to my doctor about a problem I could not solve, he said, finally, after listening carefully, "Joyce, just don't think about it."

"Sir?" I questioned.

"That's right," he said. "Don't think about it. We can think of only one thing at a time. When you start thinking about this, immediately start thinking about something else. Try this to see whether it works."

It does work!

John Milton, in PARADISE LOST, wrote:

"The mind in its own place and in
    itself
Can make a heav'n of hell, a hell of
    heav'n."

7. Consider the motive behind unkind, cruel remarks.
   Consider the pain of these:

   > I heard you lost your job.
   > When are you going on a diet?
   > When are you going to get your acne treated?
   > You could really be successful if you could only get
   > help with your wardrobe planning.

   Is the motive jealousy? insecurity? Is the person really trying to help and does not know how? Is the person making this remark because he simply does not know how to behave, because he is not socially aware of etiquette, good manners, and the Golden Rule?

   Consider the person. Consider the motive. Consider the physical, emotional, and spiritual condition of the person.

   One can respond in several ways:

   1. Smile.
   2. Smile and walk away.
   3. Acknowledge the remark and ask whether the person has suggestions for a doctor, a diet, or a certain medicine.
   4. Quietly say: "I never dreamed that you noticed. All of us have problems. I am working on mine." Ann Landers and Dear Abby suggest saying, "Why did you ask?"

   Above all, avoid sarcasm and temper, as well as crying or screaming. Remain in control. Remember that people are people. We must expect the worst at times.

8. Talk to a friend.

   Someone has said, "The best way to deal with a

problem is to talk it over with people you can trust
absolutely: God, yourself, and a friend.''

An Arabian proverb states:

> "A friend is one to whom one may pour out all the
> contents of one's heart, chaff and grain together,
> knowing that the gentlest of hands will take and sift it,
> keeping what is worth keeping, and with the breath of
> kindness, blow the rest away."

9. Relax as much as possible and let go of your stress.

You can relax. Learn to quieten your mind.
Think. Think "thoughtfully." Think reasonably.
Think rationally. For years, the drop side of snow
signs beside roads in North Carolina said "Think."
What a challenge to motorists. What a challenge to
life. Seek stillness, silence, peace, quietude. Rise
above tension.

10. Love your enemies.

This may seem to contradict the "passing-from-
out-of-the-midst-of" idea. Not at all! We love the
soul of the thief, the murderer, the slanderer. We
love with hope and a prayer. We are all created by
God in His image. Never forget that.

Ann Landers wrote:

> "When Jesus said, 'Love your enemies,' He was not
> only preaching sound ethics, but also good mental
> health. Hate is corrosive and destructive. It can ruin your
> good looks. We all know people whose inability to for-
> give — especially women who have been dumped by
> lovers or husbands — causes them to look angry or
> bitter. The agony and hostility show on their faces. They
> look defeated and sullen, hard and unsmiling. Their eyes
> are dead: their jaws are set. Their heads are down: their
> shoulders slump. They lack grace when they move. They

look like losers, and that's what they are. Shakespeare said it best: 'Heat not a furnace for your foe so hot that it do singe yourself.' "[1]

11. Try solitude.

Henry David Thoreau wrote: "I have never found the companion that was so companionable as solitude."

Most of us, regardless of how much we love people, our family, or our work, need to find time to be alone each day. We need to listen to our own heartbeat, our own breathing, our own drumbeat, our own thoughts. Husbands, do not be offended. Wives, do not be offended. Allow your mate quietness, aloneness, solitude, privacy. This may be achieved through reading, sitting quietly in a favorite place, exercising, jogging, walking, or meditating.

12. Watch thinking.

A truth of life is that we become what we think. If we think hate, envy, jealousy, fear, revenge, and greed, we become the living reality of these. Even before the actions begin, there are outward, visible signs of corrosion and corruption. If we think love, praise, joy, hope, faith, courage, compassion, care and concern, we become the living symbol of these.

Think thin is in in America. Let's start another worthy "in." Think health. Studies have shown that people who stay happy are more likely to stay healthy than those people who worry about becoming ill. A study at the National Institute of Public Health, Bethesda, Maryland, reported that people who appear confident of continued health and who make light of illnesses tend to be much healthier than people who fear the worst.

Horace Stewart, of Augusta College, Georgia, found that the rarely ill group was generally more self-confident, composed, realistic about life, and concerned, but not anxious, about health.

Often, it is not the size of life's problems, but how one faces them, that determines their effect on health. Doctors say that in serious illnesses such as cancer and heart attacks, patients who are optimistic recover much more rapidly than the unhappy and pessimistic.

13. Try to remember what you worried about yesterday or even last week.

Sometimes, you cannot remember.

14. Bite your tongue.

We almost never regret or worry about what we do not say. Paradoxically, say what you must.

15. Use questions instead of statements that sound like commands.

> Would you mind taking out the trash?
>
> Do you mind bringing in the milk?
>
> How about leaving your dirty socks in the hamper instead of your room?

16. Look back — and ahead.

Homer wrote in THE ILIAD: "Young men's minds are always changeable, but when an old man is concerned in a matter, he looks both before and after."

17. Might does not make right.

The mob cried: ". . . Crucify him . . ." Luke 23:21.

Remember, "There is strength in the union, even of very sorry men" (Homer, THE ILIAD).

A dying old man who had been betrayed looked up from his bed to say, "They have killed me this time, haven't they?"

The TALMUD states: "Therefore was a single man only first created, to teach thee that whosoever destroys a single soul from the children of man, Scripture charges him as though he had destroyed the whole world."

Realize that there is evil in the world. In SILAS MARNER, by George Eliot, Godfrey said of Dunstan: "Hurt? . . . He'll never be hurt — he was made to hurt other people."

Many wrongs spring from the desire for power, praise, and popularity as well as the desire for reward, recognition, and revenge.

18. Sleep heals many wounds.

Sophocles, around 405 B.C., wrote: "Sleep that masters all."

Shakespeare, in MACBETH, said:

> "Sleep that knits up the ravel'd sleave (sic) of care,
> The death of each day's life, sore labour's bath,
> Balm of hurt minds, great nature's second course,
> Chief nourisher in life's feast."[2]

Sleep is a great healer. We often see problems in a new perspective after a good night's rest.

Psalm 30:5 says: ". . . Weeping may endure for a night, but joy cometh in the morning."

19. Take a day off.

Our society has not yet accepted the phone call that says: "I'm depressed and tired. I'm taking the day off.'' Flu, fever, colds, viruses, yes. But fatigue, depression, boredom, no!

Once in a long, long time, if you must, take a day off. Do anything that makes you really happy: sleep, eat, travel, cry, pray, meditate, jog, shop, hunt, fish, swim, walk in the woods, visit a friend—anything! Be human.

(By the way, I have never tried this idea of skipping work, but I think it might be fun.)

20. Remember, often, ''If you circumvent the four possible ways by which a procedure can go wrong, a fifth way will promptly develop.'' (Author Unknown)

21. Let us not sell our souls or friends or character or reputation for ''thirty pieces of silver'' (Matthew 26:15).

    With obsession for possessions, for wealth, for fame, for glory, to do so is a greater temptation than one might like to believe.

22. Love people.

    Teach them gently, if you will, and patiently, if you can, but let them be free.

    Much pain, stress, and distress come from trying to change people. Henry David Thoreau probably said it best.

> ''Why should we be
>   in such desperate haste to succeed,
>   and in such desperate enterprises?
> If a man does not keep pace
>   with his companions,
>   perhaps it is because he hears
>   a different drummer.

> Let him step
>   to the music which he hears
>   however measured
>   or far away."

23. "God grant me the serenity to accept the things I cannot change . . . courage to change the things I can . . . and the wisdom to know the difference."

   Reinhold Niebuhr

24. "If we can't be thankful for what we receive, we should be thankful for what we escape."

   Arnold H. Glascow

25. "Who never has suffered, he has lived but half;
   Who never failed, he never strove or sought;
   Who never wept is stranger to a laugh,
   And he who never doubted never thought."

   J. B. Goode

26. Avoid labeling people:

> "In men whom men condemn as ill
> I find so much of goodness still.
> In men whom men pronounce divine
> I find so much of sin and blot.
> I do not dare to draw the line
> Between the two where God has not."

   Joaquin Miller

27. We shall reap the seed of our patience and our prayers, if we endure.

> "There is a destiny that makes us brothers
>   None goes his way alone,
> All that we send into the lives of others
>   Comes back into our own.

   Edwin Markham

28. Life is important, but it is not all.

"Life is the soul's nursery — its training place for the destinies of eternity."

William Thackeray

29. Sometimes, we need to consider changing.

"God comforts us
    not by changing the circumstances
    of our lives
But by changing our attitude toward them."

Author Unknown

30. Murphy's Law or the Optimist Creed is worthy of consideration.

"Nothing is as easy as it looks.
    Everything takes longer than you expect
    And if anything can go wrong — it will
    at the worst possible moment."

Life is like that!

31. Problems are traumatic, but sometimes, some of them may be solved by this thought:

Old Hogan's Goat

Old Hogan's goat was feeling fine,
Ate six red shirts from off the line;
Old Hogan grabbed him by the back
And tied him to the railroad track.
Now when the train came into sight
That goat grew pale and green with fright;
He heaved a sigh, as if in pain,
Coughed up those shirts and flagged the train.

Author Unknown

If you pick a lemon, make lemonade.

32. Do what you can, but leave the final answer to God:

"I learn as the years roll onward

And leave the past behind
That much I have counted sorrow
But proves that God is kind.
That many a flower I had longed for
Had hidden a thorn of pain
And many a rugged bypath
Led to fields of golden grain."

Author Unknown

33. Fatigue and weariness cause many problems.
Again, learn to rest, sleep, relax, and meditate.

34. Forget and forgive.

"Forget the slander you have heard,
Forget the hasty, unkind word;
Forget the quarrel, and the cause,
Forget the whole affair, because
Forgetting is the only way.
Forget the storm of yesterday . . .
Forget you're not a millionaire
Forget the gray streaks in your hair.
Forget the coffee when it's cold
Forget to kick, forget to scold.
Forget the plumber's awful charge
Forget the iceman's bill is large.
Forget the coal man and his ways
Forget the winter's blustery days.

Author Unknown

35. Slow Me Down, Lord

Slow me down, Lord

Ease the pounding of my heart
by the quieting of my mind.

Steady my hurried pace
with a vision of the eternal reach of time.

Give me, amid the confusion of the day
the calmness of the everlasting hills.

Break the tension of my nerves and muscles
with the soothing music
of the singing streams that live in my memory.

Help me to know
the magical, restoring power of sleep.

Teach me the art
of taking minute vacations
of slowing to look at a flower
to chat with a friend
to pat a dog
to read a few lines from a good book.

Slow me down, Lord

And inspire me
to send my roots deep into the soil of life's enduring values
that I may grow toward the stars
of my greater destiny.

Wilferd A. Peterson[3]

36. Living one day at a time is practical philosophy.

Just for Today

Just for today

I will live through the next twelve hours
and not tackle my whole life at once.

Just for today

I will improve my mind.
I will learn something useful.
I will read something that requires effort,
concentration.

Just for today

I will be agreeable
I will look my best
speak in a well-modulated voice
and be courteous and considerate.

Just for today

I will not find fault with friend, relative, or colleague.

I will not try to change or improve anyone but myself.

Just for today
I will have a program.
I might not follow it exactly, but I will have it.
I will save myself from two enemies — hurry and
  indecision.

Just for today
I will exercise my character in three ways:
  I will do a good turn and keep it a secret
  If anyone finds out, it won't count.

Just for today
I will do two things I don't want to do just for exercise.

Just for today
I will be unafraid.
Especially will I be unafraid to enjoy what is beautiful
And believe that as I give to the world, the world will
  give to me.

Anonymous

Compliments of
Tarmac, Inc.
71 North Market Street
Asheville, N.C.

37. The following is distributed by the Wilson County
Mental Health Association, as well as other Mental
Health groups in North Carolina. As we attempt to
escape our problems for a few minutes, or to enjoy
life, these twenty-five ideas are winners.

25 Ways to Brighten Your Days

Let yourself make a mistake
Take a walk with a friend
Give someone a present
Ask a favor of a friend
Watch children play
Sing in the shower
Do one thing well
Bake some bread
Laugh out loud
Take a risk
Slow down
Listen
Spruce up
Cry a little
Hug a child
Break a habit
Pamper yourself
Exercise a talent
Pay a compliment
Watch the sun rise
Learn something new
Do something that's hard
Encourage a young person
Treat the family like company[4]

38. Remember, sometimes, in life, it will be dark, and we cannot do much to change it.

When the lights go out, it is dark, especially if it is midnight and there are no stars and no moon!

We come to bends in the road, to curves, to

turns, and we slow down. We come to stops, and we must stop.

Sometimes, we make the wrong turn, and we must find a way and a place to turn around.

Divorce, disease, death. Accidents, wrong decisions, frustrated efforts. All cause the lights to go out. But "joy cometh in the morning" (Psalm 30:5). The sun always rises. Clouds may hinder the brightness, but light comes again.

In the physical world, as well as the emotional, there is not much we can do to keep the lights from going out. Storms come, fuses blow, accidents happen.

Did I say elsewhere in this book that I have heard my dad say many times that he believes that anyone can make a mistake in marriage just as one makes a mistake in the choice of a profession or a piece of land or in any other human effort?

Mistakes make us human. They make us all one size. Three truths: we are born, we live, we die. Another dimension: we are fallible.

But the simple question with the long answer is this: "What do I do when the lights go out, when darkness comes?"

This chapter attempts to answer that all-important question.

But you have to act immediately for a temporary solution. The answer simplified: You light one small candle and wait for the dawn.

As you reflect in the darkness, determine what has happened, and why, if you can. Say over and over, "Even this shall pass away," and say again and again, "I did the best I knew at the moment."

As a young man, before his conversion on the road to Damascus, Paul persecuted the Jews. He thought he was doing what was right. He was sincere, but Bible scholars tell us that he was sincerely wrong.

Sometimes we are sincerely wrong.

But we do the best we can in our human way.

Or, at least, that should be our goal.

One determination is this: not to blame ourselves for the errors and mistakes of others beyond what is reasonable and in keeping with good mental health. We can only carry our part of the burden. Do not think that others are infallible. On the other hand, do not blame others, beyond reason, for what happens.

It is dark when the lights go out. Do what you can. Check the fuses. Light one tiny candle. Be quiet and still and seek an answer if action will not help at the moment. Wait for the dawn. It will come . . .

39. Perhaps Ann Landers' essay entitled "Who Is Mentally Healthy?" will help us in the hour of trouble:

> Mental health, like physical health, is a dynamic, ever-changing condition. Some days you are bound to be in better shape than others. The mentally healthy person does not experience wide personality swings — on the moon one day and in the dumps the next. He has the qualities of sameness and predictability.
>
> Mentally healthy people think well of themselves. They do not waste time and energy worrying if every hair is in place, or if they made a favorable impression on Miss or Mr. X., or if they used the right fork or wore the right dress.

On occasion when every hair is not in place, or they may have used the wrong fork or worn the wrong dress, they don't agonize over it. They have a good sense of priorities and a sense of what is really important.

Mentally healthy people are able to accept the inadequacies and shortcomings of others. They do not feel the need to overhaul everyone who does not fit into the mold they have decided is "correct." They are satisfied to live and let live.

Mentally healthy people are able to accept whatever life visits upon them without going to pieces. This means financial reverses, illness, death, divorce, separation, unrequited love — the list is endless. And they have the ability to withstand the cruelties and inequities of life, to regroup, re-energize, think their way through a problem and go forward in a positive, constructive way.[5]

40. It is not the critic that counts, but the courage and suffering of the one who is in the arena, trying to win. Consider these words from "The Courage to Act," by an unknown writer.

> "It is not the critic who counts, not the man who points out how the strong man stumbled, or where the doer of deeds could have done better. The credit belongs to the man who is actually in the arena, whose face is marred by dust and sweat and blood, who strives valiantly, who errs and comes short again and again — who knows the great enthusiasm, the great devotions, and spends himself in a worthy cause, who, at the best, knows in the end the triumph of high achievements, and, who, at the worst, if he fails, at least fails while daring greatly so that his place shall never be with those cold and timid souls who know neither victory nor defeat."[6]

41. The final, all-important consideration in problem solving is God.

Ralph Waldo Emerson wrote: "Great men are

they who see that spiritual is stronger than any natural force . . .''

Alfred Tennyson said it this way:

> ''More things are wrought by prayer
> Than this world dreams of. Wherefore let thy voice
> Rise like a fountain for me night and day.
> For what are men better than sheep or goats,
> That nourish a blind life within the brain.
> If, knowing God, they lift not hands of prayer
> Both for themselves and those who call them friend?
> For so the whole round earth is every way
> Bound by gold chains about the feet of God.''

I recall the title of a book by Robert V. Ozment, released by the Fleming Revell Company in 1962: BUT GOD CAN. Even though heaven helps those who help themselves — and we must do all we can to solve our problems — we must always remember, ''But God Can!'' I remember the little chorus from Bible School, ''God Can Do Anything, Anything, Anything: God Can Do Anything But Fail!''

So often, we see lists of Scripture which can be read for certain needs. The Bible promises: ''God is our refuge and strength, a very present help in trouble'' (Psalm 46:1).

When in sorrow	John 14
When men fail you	Psalm 27
When you worry	Matthew 6:19-34
When you are in danger	Psalm 91
When you are discouraged	Isaiah 40
When doubts come	John 7:17
When you are lonely	Psalm 33 or Psalm 23
When you need courage	Joshua 1
When you grow bitter	I Corinthians 13

When you want peace	Matthew 11:25-30
When you want assurance	Romans 8:1-30
When you have sinned	Psalm 51

Answers to problems can be found

In four words: Have faith in God . . . (Mark 11:22)

In three words: Come unto me . . . (Matthew 11:28)

In two words: Seek Him . . . (Proverbs 8:17)

In one word: Pray . . . (I Thessalonians 5:17)

Chapter 15

What Is Really Important Anyway?

A universal recognition is that group of words known as "The Seven Deadly Sins": pride, envy, anger, sloth, avarice, gluttony, and lust. Ann Landers chose envy as the worst of the seven:

> "It eats you up, makes you miserable. It is petty, self-destructive, an embarrassment to your friends, and a triumph to your enemies. The most insidious aspect of envy is that it keeps you from appreciating what you have. And it poisons the well-being of your personality — because it shows."[1]

Too often we dismiss the attributes of honesty, trust, honor, and industriousness as simplistic or trite.

Mahatma Gandhi had a list of seven sins:

1. Wealth without work
2. Pleasure without conscience
3. Knowledge without character
4. Commerce without morality
5. Science without humanity
6. Worship without sacrifice
7. Politics without principle

Wealth, pleasure, knowledge, commerce, science, worship, and politics are realities of life, but they must be tempered with hard work, a clear conscience, good character, acceptable morality, love of humanity, willing sacrifice, and sound principles.

Confucius wrote: "To be able to practice five things everywhere under heaven constitutes perfect virtue . . . gravity, generosity of the soul, sincerity, earnestness, and kindness."[2] He also wrote: "There are three things which the superior man guards against: In youth . . . lust. When he is strong . . . quarrelsomeness. When he is old . . . covetousness."

> "Wanted — men.
> Not systems fit and wise
> Not faith with rigid eyes
> Not wealth in mountain piles
> Not power with gracious smiles
> Not even the potent pen —
> Wanted — men.   Author Unknown

> ". . . To win the respect of intelligent people and the affection of children; to earn the appreciation of honest critics and endure the betrayal of false friends; to appreciate beauty; to find the best in others; to leave the world a bit better, whether by a healthy child, a garden patch, or a redeemed social condition; to know that even one life has breathed easier because you lived. This is to have succeeded."
> Harry Emerson Fosdick

"We must stand for something, lest we stand for nothing" is a worthy quotation, full of truth.

In consideration of values, let us guard against false vanity. Remember: "A good leg will fail. A straight back will stoop. A black beard will turn white. A curled pate will grow bald. A fair face will wither. A full eye will wax hollow. But a good heart is the sun and the moon, for it shines bright and never changes, but keeps its course truly." William Shakespeare[3]

My mother, a sixth-grade teacher during the war years, was a lover of beautiful words. Each Sunday we clipped Blanch Manor's philosophical-poetic column, "Chatter," from THE NEWS AND OBSERVER. She always required her students to memorize the great classic poems such as Rudyard Kipling's "L'Envoi," John Greenleaf Whittier's "The Barefoot Boy," Henry Wadsworth Longfellow's "The Builders," Alfred Tennyson's "Crossing the Bar," Henry Holcomb Bennett's "The Flag Goes By," Sam Walter Foss's "House by the Side of the Road," Rudyard Kipling's "If," and Henry Wadsworth Longfellow's "Psalm of Life."

Exemplary of the beauty and power of the others, consider these lines of courage in the hour of trouble from "Invictus," by William Ernest Henley;

"Out of the night that covers me,
  Black as the Pit from pole to pole,
I thank whatever gods may be
  For my unconquerable soul.

In the fell clutch of circumstance
  I have not winced or cried aloud.
Under the bludgeonings of chance
  My head is bloody, but unbowed.

Beyond this place of wrath and tears
  Looms but the horror of the shade,
And yet the menace of the years
  Finds, and shall find me, unafraid.

It matters not how strait the gate,
  How charged with punishments the scroll,
I am the master of my fate;
  I am the captain of my soul."

In a different mood, nothing is more powerful than the words of Rudyard Kipling's "If," when he expresses such thoughts as "If you can keep your head when all about you are losing theirs and blaming it on you . . . If you can bear to hear the truth you've spoken twisted by knaves to make a trap for fools . . . Or watch the things you gave your life to, broken, and stoop to build 'em up with worn-out tools."

The beauty, the power of words! The beauty, the power of human lives! The beauty, the power of human minds!

Something that we call the soul is all that time passes on to eternity. The aim of life is to perfect and to purify the soul. This is accomplished through study and thought, tears and trials, work and struggle, faith and discipline.

The noble thoughts of the sages of the ages offer us wisdom and strength, and they may offer us part of the answer to that all-important question: "What is really important anyway?"

Part II

EXTERNAL BEAUTY

You Are Not Just A Body — You Are Somebody

Chapter 16

The Pursuit of Excellence

At a recent antique show, I saw a friend that I had not seen for a long time. She looked just as I had remembered her during my childhood. When I mentioned this fact to her, she said, "I work on it."

I remember the televison interview with Totie Fields. In consideration of all her pain and suffering, the interviewer asked her how she managed to smile and stay in such good spirits. She replied, "I work on it."

And so it is. Anything that we want, we work on it — and that includes beauty.

> We cleanse our faces faithfully, daily, or more often.
> We file our nails.
> We shampoo our hair.
> We shave our legs.
> We use deodorants daily.
> We rest.
> We sleep.
> We eat right.
> We think right.
> We find time for ourselves.
> We jog.

We exercise.
We brush our teeth.
We take time to put on makeup.
We remember to take our vitamins.
We think positively.
When we begin to think negatively, we train ourselves to think positively. And we can think only one thing and one way at a time.
We think thin when we diet.
We think hope when we cry.
We think sunshine when it rains.

There is truth in the thought that we find time to do what we want to do.

Beauty, good health, and charm require time, effort, and self-discipline. They involve the pursuit of excellence.

In manners, in business, in matters of living, think of three EEE's to symbolize the thought, "Excellence requires extra effort."

Achievement, growth, and change require conscientious, even sacrificial, effort. Dieting, exercising, and disciplining toward excellence are successful realities only to the faithful few.

In all worthy endeavors, determine to put the plus in excellence.

Another favorite thought is "Beware and be aware." Beware of the pitfalls and be aware of the pitfalls in all efforts toward self-improvement and change.

Winston Churchill wrote: "Courage is the first of human qualities because it is the quality which guarantees all others."

Often, we use the expression, V.I.P.: very important person.

V.I.P. can easily represent thoughts in efforts toward

self-esteem, self-actualization, and self-improvement.

Consider "V" for *vision*. It has been said that "a dream without a waking vision is lost."

We must plan, dream, think, determine, envision what we want to become. Draw on the subconscious, the superconscious, as some have referred to it. Those individuals who have achieved beyond the ordinary are not super-beings. They are merely human beings who have sought depth and strength from thought, determination, and indescribable effort. Ralph Waldo Emerson talked about transcendentalism — the philosophy that man, through thought, study, and effort could transcend himself and come in contact with Divine Truth. This I believe.

John Oxenham, English novelist and poet, 1852-1941, expressed the pursuit of excellence in his poem, "The Ways," quoted here in its original form:

> "To every man there openeth
>   A Way, and Ways and a Way.
>   And the High Soul climbs the High Way,
>   And the Low Soul gropes the Low,
>   And in between on the misty flats,
>   The rest drift to and fro.
>   But to every man there openeth
>   A high Way, and a Low,
>   And every man decideth
>   The Way his soul shall go."

The "I" of V.I.P. could easily represent *initiative*. "Get up and go" and "Get up and do" are all important. The longest journey starts with a single mile. Life itself begins with one stumbling step. Energy and action are key words.

Finally, all effort toward self-improvement and the

pursuit of excellence involve *proper perspective,* the "P" of V.I.P. We must not lose our sense of values. First things must always come first. What shall it be? "God, others, self." "God, self, others." "God, self, others, things." But always God. Perhaps the all-important thought is "In all thy ways acknowledge him, and he shall direct thy paths" (Proverbs 3:6).

Chapter 17

Charm

Charm is perhaps one of the most misunderstood words in the world. It implies that which is artificial, shallow, unrealistic, and even repulsive. It implies a false manner or way.

Real charm is neither of these.

Charm is simply good manners. It is doing common things uncommonly well. It is poise, respect, calm, quiet.

The universal, yet unanswered question, is "What makes a woman beautiful? charming?"

Charm is a beautiful voice, not artificial or intentionally sexy, but well-modulated, clear, relaxed.

Charm is graceful carriage, a straight spine, head high, not because of false pride, but from self-confidence that comes from having perfected those attributes which one knows to be worthy.

Charm is a sincere smile.

Charm is intensity of feeling.

Charm is a genuine interest in others.

Charm is loyalty.

Charm is love at its best.

Charm is trust.
Charm is intelligence blended with common sense.
Charm is inner class and style, not just obvious looks.
Charm is a positive attitude of confidence.
Charm is quiet dignity.
Charm is elegance of movement, of expression, of action.

Someone has said: "A beautiful woman is one I notice. A charming woman is one who notices me."

Lee Meriwether, Miss America of 1955, said: "Start from the inside and the outside will take care of itself. I am basically a happy person. And I feel that when you are feeling good inside, you have to feel right with the world — and it shows."

Socrates wrote: "I pray, Thee, O God, that I may be beautiful within."

Charm, in its purest form, is beautiful.

Beauty and charm are interrelated.

Roget's THESAURUS OF ENGLISH WORDS AND PHRASES lists these words related to beauty:

> "845. Beauty.-N. beauty, the beautiful, *le beau ideal,* loveliness . . .
> "form, elegance, grace, beauty unadorned, symmetry . . . comeliness, fairness . . . pulchritude, polish, gloss; good effect, good looks . . . bloom, brilliancy, radiance, splendour, gorgeousness, magnificence, sublimity, sublimification . . ."

Any thoughts concerning charm would be incomplete without James Barrie's famous quotation on charm:

> "It's sort of a bloom on a woman. If you have it, you don't need to have anything else, and if you don't have it, it doesn't matter what else you have. Some women, the few, have charm for all; and most have charm for one. But some have charm for none . . ."
> From WHAT EVERY WOMAN KNOWS
> Act 1

Perhaps this thought from an unknown writer expresses the best thought:

> "People are like stained-glass windows. They glow and sparkle when it is sunny and bright, but when the sun goes down, their true beauty is revealed only if there is light from within."
>
> Author Unknown

Chapter 18

What Is Class?

A young celebrity, interviewed on television concerning an impending controversial personal matter, was asked how her son would react to the adverse publicity. "He will not react," she replied. "He loves me."

"And how do you think his friends will react?" she was asked.

"I approached him about this, too, and he replied, 'Don't worry, Mom. My friends won't say anything: they have class.' "

This is an answer, a word, I have been searching for all my life — *class*. What is class? Your answer is as good as mine. But I would say that class is dignity, respect, consideration, depth, polish, humility, quietness, refinement, restraint. Class is refraining from passing judgment, restraint in speaking, discussing, gossiping.

When we look at life realistically, we know that all persons have not found that beautiful spark in their lives. Does not every town, city, community have that person or family that is known as gossipers or gossip-mongers? As children, we soon learned to avoid these persons, and if forced into their presence, we were to be careful what we said and challenged to avoid repeating what we heard. If there was a rumor in the community, someone would say, "Go ask a certain person: she will know."

How pathetic. In all of God's beauty, to be known as a gossipmonger.

A gossipmonger lacks class.

The Bible teaches: "Judge not that ye be not judged" (Matthew 7:1). Yet, God gives to us common sense and reasoning ability to see evil and wrongdoing.

Which Are You?

I watched them tearing a building down,
A gang of men in a busy town;
With a ho-heave-ho and a lusty yell
They swung a beam and the sidewalk fell.
I asked the foreman: "Are these men skilled,
And the men you'd hire if you had to build?
He gave a laugh and said, "No, indeed!
Just common labor is all I need.
I can easily wreck in a day or two,
What builders have taken a year to do."

And I thought to myself as I went on my way,
Which of these roles have I tried to play?
Am I a builder who works with care
Measuring life by the rule and square?
Am I shaping my deeds in a well-made plan,
Patiently doing the best I can?
Or am I a wrecker who walks the town,
Content with the labor of tearing down?

Unknown

Words

Boys flying kites haul in their white-winged birds
You can't do that when you're flying words.
"Careful with fire," is good advice, you know.
"Careful with words" is ten times doubly so.
Thoughts unexpressed may sometimes fall back dead,
But God himself can't kill them when they're said!

Unknown

A person with class learns the facts before
he speaks. Then he does not speak at all unless
necessary.

A person with class learns and believes the truth.
Then he does not judge.

A person with class thinks before he speaks. Concerning a
neighbor, my dad remarked that he felt that the neighbor
seldom spoke without serious thinking or forethought.

Another attribute of class is a grateful heart.

Cicero wrote: "A thankful heart is the parent of all virtues."

James Henry Potts expressed it in this way:

"Gratitude is a becoming trait. It sweetens life, cements the
bonds of friendship, gives cheer to fellowship, and makes
benevolence a joy."

Someone has said: "Do not expect gratitude. If you do, you
will lead a disappointed life."

The family is the most neglected element of gratitude.
Close friends that one sees everyday are another. We
say "thank you" quickly and methodically and think
that that is sufficient — and maybe it often is and should
be. In speaking of family and friends, Anne Morrow
Lindbergh said: "One can never pay in gratitude. One
can only pay 'in kind' somewhere else in life." We can
never pay or repay parents. The only thing we can do is

to live good, honorable, noble lives of service, passing our blessings and knowledge to others. But we can say, without hesitancy or embarrassment, "I love you, I appreciate you, I am proud of you."

Suppose you are inspired to buy a friend a birthday gift or even a friendship gift. Excitement and anticipation rise. You dress, drive your car into town, search in several stores for the perfect gift, finally find it, purchase it, and then decide that it must be wrapped perfectly, professionally, even at additional cost.

Excited, you drive to the friend's home. She is not at home. So you leave the gift inside the storm door for safety.

Days pass. You begin to worry that the gift was stolen or misplaced.

So you call. At first, you talk informally, waiting to see whether the person mentions having received the gift. Finally, the friend says: "By the way, thanks for the surprise gift. I meant to write or call, but . . ."

You eventually hang up the phone, relieved that the gift was received.

Gratitude alone does not give us class, but we cannot have class without expressed gratitude.

In addition to gratitude, there is another word that can be associated with class. That word is *magnanimity* or *magnanimous*.

> "Magnanimity: . . . loftiness of spirit enabling one to bear trouble calmly, to disdain meanness and revenge, and to make sacrifices for worthy ends . . ."

> "Magnanimous: 1. showing or suggesting a lofty or courageous spirit 2. showing or suggesting nobility of feeling and generosity of mind: forgiving . . ."
>
> From WEBSTER'S SEVENTH
> NEW COLLEGIATE DICTIONARY

A very special student friend said that she wanted me to attend her wedding and to participate. I planned to do so. As the time of the wedding approached, I realized that I could not attend. I called the student and said simply, "For personal reasons, I cannot attend your wedding. I know that you will understand."

She never questioned.

"I am sorry," she said. "If you are not all right, let me know if I can help . . . I will get someone else to do the part planned for you."

She has written, visited, and kept in touch by telephone, but we have never discussed my not attending the wedding. No one has ever exemplified a more magnanimous spirit than she.

One should let other people do what they choose, but separate oneself from that which is impossible, unbecoming, or unacceptable. This is freedom to give and to receive, to be or not to be, to do or not to do.

To seek revenge by action or indifference is truly despicable. Judging friends by denying them the freedom to make decisions and choices based on what they think is best is to try to play God concerning the happiness and destiny of others.

Magnanimity does not give us class, but one cannot have class without a magnanimous spirit.

Many think that having "class" is living in beautiful homes, driving expensive cars, and wearing elegant clothes. Maybe these are worthy, but they must walk hand in hand with other all-important attributes to make one a truly beautiful person.

Chapter 19

Serenity

Enthusiasm, energy, and vivaciousness are worthy, but serenity is the crowning glory of the mature woman. Maturity and refinement walk hand in hand with serenity. Think now of those quiet, serene, peaceful persons that you have known, not fakers or false-charmers or superficials, but genuinely-calm spirits who draw poise and quiet from inward confidence and security.

As a teenager and as a young woman, I suffered much because of misconceived ideas concerning personality and beauty. Although basically a very shy person, my "environment" led me to believe that loud, yelling, laughing, noisy persons were the ones who really had personality. One was even supposed to be clever, smart, even a bit aggressive and sarcastic, to have a "good" personality. Also, I remember being verbally reminded of the loveliness of a certain blond's hair, the perfect beauty of another's natural curls, and the "marvelous" personality of certain peers. I had no discernible, describable personality, as my "world" demanded. I had ugly, straight hair. I was a loser in every area.

Yet, there were those quiet, mature people who seemed to have serenity: teachers, mothers, ministers, ministers' wives, doctors, and even older aunts and cousins. I wanted to be like them.

The world clamors for praise, attention, and recognition. Noise is one way to get these, temporarily.

If I had advice for young girls, I would express this dream: Be healthy, be strong, be "alive," alert, energetic, enthusiastic, and vivacious, but be so in a serene, sincere, feminine way. Is this contradictory? Not at all. It is a possible dream that can come true.

Again, let us avoid superficiality and artificiality. Let us strive for depth that comes from truth and genuineness of soul. Let us be what God created us to be — in His image. Can you imagine Christ as a loud, laughing, boisterous person who sought the center of attention and wanted to be seen or heard?

How does one achieve serenity?

1. One thinks about it, dreams about it, works on it.
2. One forgets about praise, recognition, and success. What is the quotation about the butterfly? If you chase it, it will flee. If you move quietly and calmly, it may come to light upon you. Specifically, Nathaniel Hawthorne said it this way: "Happiness is a butterfly, which when pursued, is always beyond our grasp, but which, if you sit down quietly, may light upon you." Success is like that, too.

   Maybe these lines from Henry Wadsworth Longfellow's "Psalm of Life," will inspire us toward nobility, honest toil, and pure motives:

   > "Not enjoyment and not sorrow
   > Is our destined end or way,
   > But to act that each tomorrow

> Find us farther than today.
> Let us then be up and doing
>   With a heart for any fate;
>   Still achieving, still pursuing
>   Learn to labor and to wait."

A woman watched a friend receive recognition in an organization for services of several decades. Immediately, the desire for praise motivated the observing person to imitate the winning person in every way — even to the point of obvious aggression. She volunteered for every committee, every program, every chairmanship, even the presidency. The woman eventually became quite ill, physically and emotionally. She had tried, in vain, to achieve in one year what another had done quietly, unaware, over decades.

Usually, it takes a lifetime to succeed. It takes years to grow, to serve, to prove oneself worthy as one is "tested in the fires of time."

Do not work for praise or recognition; it destroys serenity. Just work and wait and pray. The reward will come one day, unaware, even if in eternity. Abraham Lincoln once said something about getting ready and waiting, that maybe someday his chance would come — and it did.

Helen Hayes said that her mother drew a distinction between achievement and success. She advised her that "achievement is the knowledge that you have studied and done the best that is in you. Success is being praised by others, and that's nice, too, but not so important or satisfying." Always aim for achievement and forget about success.

3. Seek solitude.

> "I often return to the little hill,
>   And believe that I always will,
>   For everyone needs an old grist mill
>   Where time is standing still."
>
> Irene Smith Heyman

> "Each one must make
>   a quiet place
>   within his heart
>   where he may go
>   to find himself,
>   And for a space
>   drink deeply
>   where still waters flow.
>
> Inge Gibson Caldwell

4. Enjoy what you have.

   A lesson from my ninth-grade civics class: Our wants are never satisfied. We get our wants from other people. Our wants are constantly changing.

   Someone has said that we are rich in proportion to the things that we are able to do without.

   Epictetus wrote: "Contentment consists not in great wealth, but in few wants."

5. Realize that early death and disease are often linked to lack of serenity.

6. If loud, aggressive personalities trouble you, avoid them whenever possible.

7. Do the best you can and leave the results to a Power higher than yourself.

Chapter 20

Silence

As a child, I thought that she was the prettiest person that I had ever seen. One day, an older person commented that she was pretty until she spoke. Later, I realized the truth of her statement. When I became older, I realized that the tone of voice, choice of words, pronunciation, and attitudes implied by her speech distracted.

George Bernard Shaw, in PYGMALION, (Broadway's MY FAIR LADY), created a lady from Liza, basically, by teaching her to speak beautifully.

Learning to speak beautifully is another chapter.

There is beauty in knowing when not to speak at all. There is beauty in silence.

RULE OF LIFE recorded this: "Of all virtues, Zeno made choice of silence; for by it, said he, 'I hear other men's imperfections and conceal my own.' "

Practice silence when dealing with enemies.

"Euripides was wont to say that silence was an answer to a wise man, but we seem to have greater occasion for it in our dealings with fools and unreasonable persons, but men of breeding and sense will be satisfied with reason and fair words."

Plutarch

"A good word is an easy obligation, but not to speak ill requires only our silence, which costs us nothing."

John Tillotson

"It is the wise head that makes the still tongue."

W. J. Lucas

"Most men speak when they do not know how to be silent. He is wise who knows when to hold his peace. Tie your tongue, lest it be wanton and luxuriate. Keep it within the banks. A rapidly flowing river soon collects mud."

Saint Ambrose

"Silence never shows itself so great an advantage as when it made the reply to calumny and defamation."

Joseph Addison

Sometimes we speak of someone's weak or vulnerable point as his Achilles' heel. In Greek mythology, Achilles was the son of mortal man, Peleus, and the sea goddess, Thetis. Upon hearing the prophecy of Achilles' death at Troy, Thetis dipped Achilles in the river Styx to make him invulnerable and to give him eternal life.

However, in holding him to dip him, she held him by the heel, and the waters did not touch that part of his body.

Achilles fought in many battles without injury. During the Trojan War, however, Paris, the prince of Troy, shot an arrow into Achilles' heel, and he died of his wound.

Everyone has a weak spot, an Achilles' heel. Let us resolve now that we will not let it be our tongue. There is a time to speak and a time to be silent.

Move peacefully and quietly if there is confusion,

noise, and haste, aware of the beauty and peace of quietness and silence.

Chapter 21

The Voice

The human voice is the messenger of the soul.

Many people who have beautiful physical bodies have become less attractive by abuse or misuse of the voice through affectation or unnaturalness of tone.

The voice can be trained. Remember French class where one was taught to put words at the tip of the tongue just at the teeth at the front of the mouth — to sound like the French? Remember voice and diction where one was taught to drop the voice low into the throat or even the chest to avoid that shrill, high-strung offense?

But the most offensive voice is the unnatural, artificial, "prissy," sophisticated tone that one develops when a so-called education "goes to one's head," one inherits or marries too much money, or visits another area of the country.

Another offensive voice is that attempt at an ultra-sexy voice, especially on the telephone.

Another pathetic circumstance is the middle-aged

woman who answers the telephone in an immature manner by trying to sound young and sexy. How embarrassing, how disgusting to an innocent caller!

Have you ever had someone to answer the phone with the sound of a snake-charming instrument made at the tip of the tongue, against the teeth, with a "Hey Lou" instead of "Hello." Sometimes, the sound is drawn out to sound "Hey Lou ou-ou" — if it were possible to write such a sound! Try this sound sometime when you are alone — and not on the phone.

Another offensive sound is "Hel loh-oh-oh" with the shrill, high-pitched, drawn-out sound. It's that "come-and-get-me-I'm-ready" sound.

After the phone is lifted to answer, hesitancy in answering so that one can "create" just the right sound is embarrassing. It is all so immature, so obvious.

We should always answer the telephone so that priest, prophet, or president would not be offended or embarrassed by our tone and accent. Never do we want a male to think, "Well, well. I didn't expect all this—" unless we want him to expect it!

A simple, quiet, cultured "hello" coming from the throat area or the chest area is all that is needed. When the caller identifies himself or herself, we, as refined people, with a degree of class and culture, can identify ourselves further if we choose to do so.

Considering further the use of the voice, we realize that there is a level of language which is beautiful, accurate, and non-artificial, when blended with a natural voice tone, that is acceptable anytime, anywhere, with anyone. We do not need to use big words or profound thoughts to fit into society or to participate in any event. A calm, natural, soft-spoken, well-thought idea will suffice and be acceptable.

Ralph Waldo Emerson wrote over one hundred years ago a truth which still inspires:

> "The sweetest music is not oratorios, but the human voice when it speaks from its instant life tones of tenderness, truth, and courage."

Chapter 22

Putting One's Best Foot Forward

As was emphasized earlier, putting the plus in excellence is a challenge in every area of life. Grooming is no exception. Consciously, or subconsciously, without stress, we should strive to be our very best in all ways and at all times.

Good grooming makes a difference. Little things mean a lot, as the aged expression says.

Consider the following wardrobe ideas:

1. Clothes that fit
2. Hemlines that are even, with no hemming thread showing on the outside
3. Sleeves and other areas free from perspiration stains as well as other blotches and soiled spots
4. Buttons well-sewn, none missing
5. Seams well-sewn, none split
6. Stockings with no runs, tears, or holes
7. Pants not too long or too short. A good rule for length: touching the top of the foot in front and one-half inch off the floor in the back or heel area
8. Shoes polished, brushed, or dusted; heels clean, recapped when worn; good soles

9. Underclothes that do not show through
10. Accessories that enhance, not distract
11. Clothes cleaned and pressed; all wrinkles "out"

Additionally:

1. Hair that is "squeaky" clean, trimmed for shape, dead or uneven ends, and with permanent or "curls" added if needed or preferred
2. Teeth clean, brushed; mouthwash; sugarfree mint
3. Eyebrows plucked from beneath for stray brows; also stray brows from above the nose between brows
4. Legs and underarms shaved or hair removed
5. Fingernails clean, trimmed, or filed
6. Underarm deodorant
7. Toenails trimmed; feet soaked to remove dead skin—and deodorized

Chapter 23

Things Not to Do If You Want to Be Appealing to the One You Love

I f you want a man to love you . . . No, let's start again. If you want to have an intimate, one-to-one, close, personal relationship with another human being of the opposite sex, consider these:

1. Smoking

   Yes, you may smoke. But smoke gets in the hair, on clothes, on the skin, in the breath — everywhere, in everything. It kills bath powder and high-priced perfume, all! So, unless one wants to risk the possibility of not "smelling" feminine, do not smoke.

2. Eating onions

   Or garlic or any other highly seasoned dressing such as French dressing or onion dip, no matter how much you like them or enjoy them. Others can smell these all day, all night, and even the next morning.

   A reader wrote the following to Dr. Lawrence E. Lamb, who writes the column, "Health," for THE WILSON DAILY TIMES:

   "Dear Dr. Lamb — When I eat something that has been spiced with garlic, I tend to have garlic breath for two to four days afterward. I can't taste it or smell it, but my husband has convinced me that it is very much there. I am very conscientious about brushing my teeth and tongue, so I don't think that is the problem. I avoid garlic when I can, but sometimes I don't know it has been used . . . I would appreciate any information you can send me."

Dr. Lamb answered:

"It is far more common than you think. Most people think that bad breath means there is some problem in their mouth — and that certainly can be one cause . . . But a surprisingly large number of people don't realize that a lot of bad breath comes from the lungs and bloodstream. Breath mints and mouth wash won't reach those odors.

"Garlic is a good example and it is similar to alcohol in this regard. The chemical that causes the scent is in your bloodstream, not in your stomach. As the blood flows to the lungs, the chemical vapor passes out with the air you exhale. That is the basis of the alcohol breath test.

"You can brush your teeth all day and it will be there from your bloodstream until the chemical causing the odor is eliminated from your body . . .

"Your best course is to avoid garlic. There is no way to hasten its elimination from your bloodstream, once it has been absorbed . . ."[1]

I wonder whether diet groups that recommend onions and garlic and other strong seasonings realize what they do to romance. Some say that the new self-image from weight loss leads to false pride which sometimes leads to divorce. It could be the garlic, not the weight loss!

A friend expected her fiancé whom she had not seen in several months. That day she chose to eat a tossed salad filled with raw onions. Eventually, she and her fiancé called off their engagement. The onions, and other similar choices at other times, may have had their effect.

3. Talking excessively

This is like an automobile horn that will not stop blowing or a siren that will not stop sounding. No one can pull the wires or kick the object. Many husbands (and wives) run!

A young woman who talked and smoked incessantly cried and cried because she and her husband were considering filing for divorce.

Some people may enjoy non-stop talkers. Most people prefer another brand!

4. Forgetting cleanliness

Cleanliness is next to godliness. One's body must always be immaculate, inside and out. A young woman confessed: "I divorced him because he did not know how to take a bath." A young man said: "I couldn't stay with her. She wasn't clean enough for me." Did you know that there are those who refuse to take a bath, or a good bath, and who refuse to brush their teeth.

This business of personal cleanliness is serious. It can make or break a marriage.

If a doctor says that daily feminine hygiene is not a must, find another doctor — or use common sense and go against what he recommends.

Intimate love is like calories. Though there are exceptions, you cannot have excessive calories and a slim body. Though there are exceptions, you cannot have intimate love mixed with smoke, onions, excessive talking, and a body that is not clean.

Chapter 24

The Face

Because makeup and cosmetics and one's face are inseparable, let us talk about face care.

Protection from the sun

A panel of experts appointed by the Food and Drug Administration recommended twenty-one ingredients in sun-screening products that help protect people from burning and reduce the risk of skin cancer. Read labels and explanations to be sure that the product you buy protects you from the sun.

The panel of experts separated people into five skin types, from those with sensitive skin that always burns easily and never tans to those whose skin rarely burns and tans profusely.

People with the most sensitive skins should use a product which they would assign the highest rating. The panel suggested that the ratings range from 2 to 8, with the numbers based on the multiples of time the preparation permits a person to remain in the sun.

For instance, a product bearing a "4" rating would permit a person to stay in the sun without getting burned four times longer than without any sunscreen. The higher the number, the greater the protection. But be careful.

The panel also recommended that all manufacturers be required to display the product rating on the label with the warning: "Overexposure to the sun may lead to premature aging of the skin and to skin cancer. The liberal and regular use of this product may reduce the chance of premature aging of the skin and skin cancer."

Because no one can remember all the difficult names of all the chemicals or ingredients used for sunscreening, be aware of the label quoted above. Amino Benzoic Acid, also called Para-Amino Benzoic Acid, better known as PABA, is perhaps the most popular — and is a good example of the difficulty of the chemicals' names. Sometimes, the labels refer to the SPF (skin protection factor).

Exercising one's face

Go ahead. Make a face. It is good for you. But do it privately, of course.

Everyone is so concerned about exercising the other parts of the body that the 52 muscles of the face are often neglected. Why jog, swim, play tennis, or cycle to keep the body in good condition and neglect a vital part of the body — the face? What's wrong with wanting to look good as well as feel good. Keeping the face in shape with the rest of the body is just another part of a person's health and well-being.

Try the following facial exercises:

A. Move the chin up, up, up, tilting the head back.
B. Try to touch the nose with the lower lip.
C. Stretch the mouth and the left side of the cheek to the right side as far as possible. Repeat with the right side.
D. Say "ee-oh" several times, involving as much action as possible in the mouth and cheeks.
E. Fill cheeks (mouth) with air by blowing. Then pretend to chew with the mouth closed.
F. Close the mouth. Pretend to cleanse or rinse with water.
G. Pretend that your nose itches. Try to twist it to relieve the itching.
H. Clinch teeth and smile. Feel neck muscles tighten.
I. Turn the head to the left. Continue to lift the chin to feel

the neck muscles as they pull. Exercise the right side in the same way.

There are other exercises which are as effective as these. Discover them by experimenting in front of a mirror. The face may even become sore for a few days, but soreness is proof of the need for exercise.

Remember, one can relax the face simply through thought and conscientious effort.

Above all, do not be afraid to wash your face, to clean your face, to exercise your face, either by planned, private exercises — or by smiling.

We read so much about the possible fragility of the face. There are those who tell us not to put water on the face, not to use soap, not to smile (it might cause wrinkles), and not to exercise. There are those who give us complexes and "nerves" and hypertension (if we really cared that much), because they declare and declare that cleaning the face by going up or down or around at the wrong time in the wrong way will cause us to age decades in one night! Please do not be misled in this way.

Let us consider the above by recalling that the face is the only part of the body that is continuously exposed to the elements. It is the only part of our body that cannot be protected, reasonably, from the rain, cold, wind, and sun. Even our hands, perhaps the most-used part of our body, can be protected much of the time.

What does this fact say to us? God did not create us as fragile dolls with fragile faces. We do not need to treat ourselves as fluffy dandelions. Caution and common sense are in order concerning face care, especially concerning the sun, but generally, soap, water, and movement are not going to ruin our skin or make us look older.

One suggestion. Through unconscious gesturing, we sometimes cause wrinkles to form across our forehead. Be careful about this, especially when putting on eye makeup, or other makeup, or when listening attentively to an interesting, or maybe surprising, conversation.

The secret of a beautiful face

The secret of a beautiful face, as well as eternal youth, is happiness. Maybe we should repeat that happiness comes from within the body to the outside of the body through the face. Just as one cannot fake a smile, one cannot fake happiness. "Watch the eyes," experts tell us, "to discern the truth." Remember the Watergate hearings?

A woman who was having marital problems laughed excessively, boisterously, and unceasingly — a nervous, artificial laugh. Psychologists label this as a cover-up for fear and unhappiness.

Robbers of facial beauty

1. Fatigue
2. Stress
3. Hate
4. Envy
5. Jealousy
6. Depression
7. Hostility
8. Anger
9. Irritability
10. Negative attitudes
11. Pessimism
12. Prejudice
13. Sun
14. Boredom

Contributors to facial beauty

1. Love
2. Faith
3. Hope

4. Peace
5. Serenity
6. Sincerity
7. Compassion
8. Smiles
9. Concern

In addition to these, proper cleansing, moisturizing, and again, exercising, enhance. Good eating habits and a balanced diet are a must. Drink plenty of water. Water "waters" the face and flushes impurities that affect the skin.

Wash the face with tap water and plenty of good soap, gently, but firmly, without pushing the skin. Then rinse thoroughly by splashing with tap water fifteen or twenty times. Apply moisturizer while the face is still damp. Thorough cleansing with Johnson's Baby Oil, or a similar product, should precede the washing and moisturizing, of course.

Water is the only moisturizer that does any good for the skin. The main purpose of moisturizing creams or lotions is to seal the greatest skin moisturizer of all-water. Again, moisturizer seals the water into the skin.

If you want a real beautifier, and a good morning awakener, splash tap water, cool or cold, on your face upon rising. It closes the pores, helps to chase swollen eyes, and gives a fresh, wide-awake look. Try it: it works!

Again, the most beautiful face is that one that glows from the beautiful person within.

Chapter 25

Cosmetics

L ike all things, use of makeup or cosmetics must be simplified. Let us see whether we can list the ABC's of makeup. Consider:

A. Application
B. Buying
C. Common sense

Concerning application: Do not be afraid of makeup. With the light, smooth, modern blends, one is not going to apply too much.

There are two exceptions:

1. Rouge—too dark and too much
2. Eyebrows—too dark and too much

One other thing: Regardless of any trends or fads or fashions, present, past, or future, if you have any true pink lipstick, or light pink lipstick, or "obvious" pink lipstick, discard it. It clashes noticeably with too many shades and colors, especially true red. Especially, if one wears red, one must be careful about the shade of lipstick worn. Consult an expert. Do not purchase an expensive name-brand dress or outfit and then cheapen it with the wrong shade or color of lipstick. Lipstick must blend with the color one wears. Of course, if one wears white or neutrals, one is freer in the choice.

Be careful about lipstick changes. I remember when very pale lipsticks were popular. A friend, in her thirties, chose to wear very pale lipstick. I thought that it made her look sick. Of course, she was free to choose what she thought was best.

But let us go back to rouge. When I was a teenager, an adult friend wore much too much rouge. When I questioned another adult about this, she replied that perhaps the woman got up before daybreak, applied the rouge, and could not really tell how much she was applying. For a long time, I believed that explanation to be true.

Do not apply too much rouge. Soften rouge with loose powder, applied with cotton. Try Johnson's Baby Powder. It works!

If rouge disintegrates, apply a little more on top of your powder. Yes, the cream kind. Or try blusher or powdered rouge. But apply more if you look pale. Put a dot of rouge, blended, on the tip of the nose and chin and forehead. It gives one a sun-kissed look. Have you ever tried lipstick for rouge and eyeshadow. It works — even if cosmetic experts panic at the thought.

Do not wear eyebrow coloring that is black and thick and exaggerated. It looks dirty and smutty and obvious. Try taupe, beige, or brown. It "shows" and works, even for dark hair.

Again, do not be afraid of makeup. I have a few friends who say that they do not need anything but a little lipstick. But most of us prefer a little more. Experiment — not on your wedding day, or the day you make that all-important speech, or the day you appear on television, but quietly, on a free Saturday, experiment with makeup in the privacy of your home.

In Ivey's self-improvement course, participants were asked to suggest one improvement for each person. Someone wrote: "Tell Sally to do something to enhance her eyes."

Sally went downstairs, bought a blue eyeliner cream stick, with the advice of a competent consultant — and changed her appearance.

Try using a darker shade of brown than your foundation between the eyelashes and the eyebrows. It might work for you. Some of us are too pale above our eyes, just under our brows.

Try a little lipstick in this area, as well as rouge. Experts will scream, as we said, but we will not hear them. We shall be at home alone, quietly experimenting.

Study ads. They help. They provide ideas for variety.

If your chin, jawline, or nose protrude, try applying a darker shade than the foundation. Blend well. This is called shading or contouring. It works.

Makeup consultants and cosmetic experts can help us.

As in all knowledge, their recommendations must be blended with common sense. For example, we are sometimes led to believe that if we apply makeup this way or that way, or too high or too low in a "prohibited" area that we will look like ghosts or clowns or ancients. This is not so. We are led to believe that for the best effect, we should apply eyeliner half way here, a fourth of the way there, and never everywhere. This is not true. Apply it. Look at yourself. You can see.

Smudge it by running your little finger gently over it. Use blue or brown or green. For most kinds, a kleenex removes it usually, if you are unhappy with the effect.

Again, if you need help beyond yourself, or if you need new makeup, go to someone you can trust. Ask. Someone will suggest to you those consultants who are capable and trustworthy.

Consider the following:

1. A good moisturizer to apply under makeup and at bedtime.
2. A foundation, cream or liquid, that blends with your skin — maybe a wee bit darker.
3. Cream rouge that blends with skin, hair, and eyes.
4. Eyeliner. Smoky eye pencils frame lashes with a background of smudgy mysteriousness and draw color from the eyes. Try it. It works.
5. Mascara. Avoid heavy black.
6. Face powder. Try Johnson's Baby Powder.
7. A cleanser. Johnson's Baby Oil is super, even for stubborn eye makeup.
8. An astringent. Dickinson's Witch Hazel cannot be "beat."
9. Foundation cream a bit darker than the overall foundation. This is for shading or contouring parts of the face such as the chin or jawline or nose — if we wish for these to recede.
10. Lip liner. A luxury that pays big dividends in appearance.
11. Light, even white, cream or stick, Use to cover circles under eyes. Apply. Smudge lightly. Let set. Then apply foundation. Works on wrinkles around the mouth, too.

Special note: Proper foundation should not only cover the skin, but enhance the complexion. A yellow-hued skin needs a foundation with a pink or peach tone. Pink skin looks best with a strictly beige tone. Grayish skin calls for peach or rose.

Americans spend over $9 billion annually on cosmetics ranging from bubblebaths to hair dyes, makeup, deodorants, tooth paste, and baby powder. Almost every one of us is a part of this.

Again, use common sense. Experiment. Find what is best for you and stick with it basically, except for minor changes for improvement occasionally. Do not be affected by every whim of fad or fashion. The natural instinct of being a woman will help you to choose wisely. Follow nature's teachings and yearnings. You cannot fail.

Finally, when you look in the mirror, do not see a face. See a canvas. See potential. Makeup can be a great costume. Consider makeup as the clothing of the face.

Chapter 26

Beauty Aid Discoveries

E ven though most of these beauty aids are mentioned elsewhere in this book, they merit space in a chapter "all their own."

1. The loofah glove, which may be purchased from such fine stores as The Emporium, North Hills, Raleigh, is nature's beauty treatment for the bath. It may seem a bit hard and incredible initially, but when softened with warm water and plenty of soap, it stimulates, cleans, and removes dead skin on elbows, feet, and other areas. It is super for bathing and stimulating the entire body and removes easily excessive deodorant that accumulates underarm or bath powder that does not seem to go away with regular bathing. Loofahs also come in squares or pads. Be sure to wash them thoroughly after each use and dry them in plenty of fresh air.

2. Johnson's Baby Powder soothes and smoothes an adult body from head to toe, giving the body a baby-soft touch. It will not interfere with perfume, cologne, or other bath powder. It is good face powder, too. It simply softens and velvetizes. Makeup shades and colors come through beautifully. Use a piece of cotton to apply. Wipe off excess.

3. Johnson's Baby Oil cleans every kind of makeup from the face, including eye makeup. Use it before the bath with excess removed by kleenex and with soap and water during the bath. It is also a good lubricant and super for wrinkles.

4. Have you ever used a twist board? This simple piece of equipment is helpful in efforts toward slenderizing the body. It is simply two squares, one 10 by 10, the other 8 x 8, with an insert which allows turning when one stands on top of the 8 x 8 board and turns the body from side to side. Be sure to hold to something sturdy in initial use to prevent falling. These can be ordered from many mail order houses.

5. A pumice stone (the *um* of pum rhymes with the *um* of rum) is excellent for removing calluses from the feet or dead skin from the heels. Be sure that any surface "buffed" is clean and dry.

6. A slant board is excellent for reversing the laws of gravity. These can be purchased or they can be built at home if one has a board about six or seven feet long, about fifteen inches wide, and which can be safely raised about twelve to eighteen inches at one end. By raising the legs higher than the head, one reverses the flow of blood, opposes gravity, and gives the body and face a lift. Swollen feet and ankles are relieved, pressure on internal organs is lightened, and scalp and complexion receive increased blood supply. Twenty minutes rest on a slant board is worth an hour's nap.

7. Dermage, a relatively new line of cosmetics, is superb. At the 1977 meeting of the American Academy of Dermatology, a group of physicians began formulating plans for a new group of cosmetics. Dermage was the result. These are "problem-free, blemish-avoiding, and elegant." They also contain sun-screen ingredients. You will need to try these to appreciate their superior quality.

8. Pantene Thickening Shampoo de Pantene for Fine or Thin Hair is superior. Because my thin, fine hair has always been a problem, the discovery of Pantene is a real joy.

9. White House Apple Cider Vinegar is a household miracle. Generally, its uses, related to beauty, involve mixing a reasonable amount of vinegar, depending on purpose, with water. For example, a teaspoon or a tablespoon, mixed with a pint of water makes a good face and body splash — an astringent to restore balance to the skin, or a few tablespoons in the bath are refreshing. A teaspoon in a glass of water, applied as a final rinse of the hair, is good. There are those who say that a teaspoon of vinegar in a glass of water, after meals, helps dissolve fat, serves as a diuretic, and aids in weight loss. If rubbed on hands, or any other part of the body, vinegar helps remove strong odors caused by onions or fish. Also, it is good for itching skin or insect bites. Because of its acid content, it is best not to use it as a mouthwash or to let it linger on one's teeth.

10. Centrum is an answer-to-prayer vitamin by Lederle. It is a "high potency multivitamin, multimineral formula, from A to Zinc," its label states. It is good for stress. Regardless of the quality of one's diet, a good vitamin supplement is a winner for most of us. The body will discard excess. Ask your doctor about this idea and this product.

   ("CENTRUM is a registered trademark of Lederle Laboratories Division, American Cyanamid Company.")

11. Noxema is an age-old joy. So often, we are fascinated by new products, but let us "not be the first by which the new is tried, nor last to lay the old aside." Noxema, as a cleanser, moisturizer, and softener, has been "tried and tested in the fires of time," and has come out with accolades and crowns.

12. Petroleum jelly or petrolatum, better known as vaseline, is excellent for wrinkles. Dr. Lawrence Lamb, in his column, "Health," wrote: "Once you have wrinkles, the only thing you can do for yourself is to use moisturizers. One of the best is petrolatum (Vaseline). The heavy oil mixture will trap moisture in your skin and cause wrinkles

to disappear. It is better than most expensive moisturizers with fancy names.

"The other choice is surgery and this can produce good results in the hands of a skilled cosmetic surgeon.

"Besides the sun, the other common factor that causes wrinkles is cigarette smoking. Women who smoke tend to have prominent crow's feet wrinkles earlier in life and often look ten years older than women who do not smoke . . ."

Chapter 27

Wardrobe—Clothes—You

I n selecting clothes, simplicity is again the key, especially in selecting a basic wardrobe.

1. First, select a basic color such as navy or black or brown and blend and coordinate. For example, with brown, one can blend beige, tan, off-white, taupe, and even shades of wine and maroon. Deep wine, or burgundy, shoes can be worn with almost everything. Taupe is almost as versatile. Black is now worn with shades of tan or brown. So is navy.

   One basic outfit in "dark neutrals" or navy can be worn for church, funerals, weddings, or any other "dress-up" occasions.

2. Remember, clothes enhance, but they do not "make the man." Poise, facial expressions, neatness, cleanliness, and attitude should dominate.

3. Simplicity is elegance: elegance is simplicity. Frills are for fun, variety, sports, or the formal. So are vivid colors. We are talking about basics.

4. We are told that color choice stems from two areas: orange, and undertones of orange; and blue and undertones of blue. Think of the colors you wear best. You will see which category is yours. Often, blonds wear shades of

orange well and brunettes, blue. Color of hair and eyes are important, but complexion is also a determining factor. Again, all colors can be traced to shades or tones of orange or blue.

5. Usually, the colors that make you feel comfortable and "pretty" are your best colors. Nature and instinct tell you. As you wear colors, people will tell you.

   But be careful. If you wear yellow, you will not be able to wear all shades of yellow effectively. Some yellows have undertones of blue; some orange. The same is true of blues. If you are a "blue" person, all shades of blue will not be becoming to you. Again, you can tell: let instinct be your guide.

   Ask reliable salespersons for opinions and ideas, even if you cannot buy. They will help you willingly, usually. That is their business, their joy, their pride.

6. Try to buy quality clothes, on sale, if possible. If you buy only one piece or one item occasionally, you will be surprised how quickly you will build a good, basic, quality wardrobe.

7. Window-shop. Study ads and observe television personalities for ideas. Glean and apply what is practical for you, but do not become overwhelmed or too greatly influenced.

8. Clean your closet. Separate summer and winter clothes. Pack in clean boxes in a clean, cool place any clothes that you have not worn for a long time. When you unpack them, or "find them" again, you will be pleased. Sometimes it is like having something new to wear. Many clothes are neglected because of boredom — not from wearing them, but from seeing them so often.

9. Though repetitive, just a reminder to take time to sew on buttons, level and repair hems, and press clothes that need this special care.

10. Be careful about line, design, and fabrics. Some materials and designs make us look larger, thinner, taller, or shorter.

11. Be sensible about hem lengths as they relate to your own

personal style and feelings. You will know when you feel chic.

12. Find your own personal style. If blazers thrill you, wear them. If heels are your joy, wear them. If blouses excite you, choose a variety. If pants are your forte, wear them to appropriate places.

Jan Jennings, writing for Copley News Service, said that "choosing the right wardrobe can give men and women a competitive edge," and "how you dress really matters in the business world."

She quoted Dr. Joan T. Werner, associate professor of sociology at San Diego State University, who teaches a course on what makes a person attractive and how clothing affects the image.

Jennings writes that "according to Werner, the woman wishing to be successful in business should be the counterpart of the male businessman in the dapper three-piece suit, tailored shirt, and tie."

"She should definitely wear a skirt, not pants," said Werner. "She should wear a tailored blouse with a nice, tailored jacket. A scarf serves the same purpose as a tie for a gentleman. And a vest is often suitable.

"She should wear neutral hosiery and high heels. The height accentuates her stature and bearing in her position. Depending upon her needs, a businesslike briefcase is important."

"Werner said that colors of attire should be subdued," according to Jennings. "Nothing flashy. No oranges, yellows, reds, or salmons. Just subtle grays, tans, browns, black, and dark blue. In a year when shades of plum are the high-fashion colors, mauve might be the right shade. Jewelry must be minimized.

"In order to be taken seriously in the business world,

you must look the part," said Warner. "That rules out sexy, flashy, or frilly numbers.

"When you show up for a business appointment or an interview, you must look like you mean business," she said.

Also, "Hair and makeup are important image builders . . . Makeup should be understated, nothing strong or garish, just enough cosmetics to accent the woman's good features and to minimize the negative features while showing that she is well-kept and in control of her appearance, as well as her business sense."

Further, Jennings quotes Werner as saying, "Basically, the woman must learn that she must dress for the occasion. It is like a uniform. It is the 'company image.' It is 'fitting in.' "

And then Jennings states a very unique, though important point, for consideration. She writes: "And that, of course, may rule out the idea of dressing to suit yourself, ignoring the rest. We wear uniforms to play tennis or golf — if we are to look the part. The same holds true in the business world. We must dress the part.

"And perhaps even more important, the woman who wishes to climb the business ladder should dress for the job she wants, not for the job she has. Look the part, be competent, and you may well get there."

The article stated further that "Werner said people who believe their personality and ability should speak for themselves may be in for rude awakenings. Even if they have achieved a degree of career success, inappropriate dress could be making their colleagues uncomfortable and could ultimately inhibit their success. . . . Personal appearance is not simply an individual concern. It is an important social phenomenon.

"Werner offers no solace to the overweight," according to Jennings. "Thin is in today," she noted. "The thinner the better. It shows discipline and control, as well as presenting an attractive, lithe, and supple body."

Finally, the article stated that "Werner said that if we face reality, we permit our clothing to be determined by our peer group, by the people with whom we work and those with whom we would like to work. We think we are individuals, but actually, we must conform to the standards of our jobs . . ."[1]

Thoughts presented by Dr. Joan Werner and Jan Jennings are worthy of consideration if one is a part of the business world.

Often, on special occasions, I have been advised and assisted concerning appropriate dress. At times, I did not feel comfortable, or "like my true self," but I did have the security of knowing that for that moment and that occasion, I was appropriately dressed.

Could we add, with understanding, that beyond the very important area of the "formal business world," freedom and femininity are essentials, and the freedom to select comfortable and appealing styles is a must? To preserve and perpetuate that unique privilege of being a girl — or a woman — is a must, even in wardrobing, clothes, costuming, or dress. Good taste and femininity are the words, not fads, high fashion, and fake.

Finally, these lines recalled from my first-grade music class:

> "Handsome is as handsome does,
>   So the wise men say,
>   Feathers fine may make fine birds,

But folks are not that way.
It's what's that's in your heart that counts,
Deny it if you can . . .
I'm not impressed with how you're dressed,
'Cause clothes don't make the man.''

Author Unknown

Chapter 28

The Essential Negatives

During World War II, a famous song began: "You've got to accentuate the positive, eliminate the negative, latch on to the affirmative . . ."[1] In being one's best self, consider:

1. After you have dressed for work or to go out during the evening, forget your appearance except for a subconscious caring or an occasional touchup. Do not finger with hair, check make-up, or pull a collar or scarf. Place all and arrange all in the best way possible — and then leave these without rearrangement.

2. In responding to a compliment, accept the compliment graciously by saying, "Thank you. Thank you very much." Alice Bell recommends a new dimension by suggesting that one add: "Thank you. You are so nice." Or "Thank you. Aren't you nice?" This turns the compliment and attention to the person who has graciously complimented you. Do not say, "Oh, this old dress. It's as old as the hills." Or "Oh, my hair, I couldn't do a thing with it this morning."

3. Do not take your troubles to work. Shakespeare coined a phrase about all of us being actors and actresses on the stage — and sometimes we must be. We must not be

insincere, but sometimes we must hide our problems and our feelings until we can find solutions or changes.

4. Similar to the above, do not wear your heart on your face unless you are happy. Was it Chaucer who described one feature of the teacher by saying that the students could discern the mood of the day by observing the expression on the teacher's face?

5. If you sell shoes and one shoe does not fit, do not say that one foot is larger. Emphasize that one foot is smaller.

   If you sell peanuts, do not put in more than one pound and then dump a few ounces. Put in less than a pound and add. A line will form at your counter — and that is good, if you are paid on commission!

6. If you are a clerk or doctor or a public employee, never reply by using the word Ma'am. Do not say, "Would there be anything else, Ma'am?" I do not know what to recommend. But women, after a certain youthful age, dislike being referred to as Ma'am.

7. Remember, put a piece of string on a table. Push it and it will go nowhere. Pull it and it will follow you wherever you go.

8. Do not be sad on Monday: it is one-seventh of your life.

9. Never tell a person he is wrong. Even if he is and realizes this, he will dislike you for the rest of his life — and yours, too. Say instead, "I thought" or "I heard" or "I read" but "I may be wrong . . ."

Chapter 29

Manners

T wo thoughts are synonymous: manners and the Golden Rule:

> Therefore all things whatsoever you would that men should do to you, do ye even so to them: for this is the law and the prophets'' (Matthew 7:12).

Manners refer to social conduct or rules of conduct acceptable according to prevalent customs.

A related idea is what we call etiquette. Etiquette, a set of rules for social occasions, is determined by experts who decide what is acceptable.

A good etiquette book is a wise investment, even though borrowing one from a library is possible and practical.

As we strive to simplify our lives toward confidence and security, knowledge of the rules of etiquette or good manners is no exception in our efforts. Because one of our most involved social functions is eating, let us consider ideas which may help us to be more at ease:

1. Sit and rise from the table from the left of your chair as you face the table.
2. Pass all food to the right, especially during first servings.
3. Cut only one or two bites of meat at the time.
4. Cut food in one direction only. Do not "saw" back and forth.
5. Pass salt and pepper together always, even though only one has been requested.
6. Eat fried chicken with the fingers on informal occasions. On more formal occasions, use a fork and knife.
7. Leave the butter knife on the butter dish and pass butter dish and knife together.
8. Put rolls and butter on the bread and butter plate, if there is one. Otherwise, use the salad plate if it is dry. Use the dinner plate, if necessary.
9. Lift food to the mouth *on* the fork whenever possible. Never push prongs into the food unless absolutely necessary. Some salads necessitate an exception.
10. Use silver from the outside in. Trust the person who set the table to tell you, in this way, which pieces to use first.
11. Notice your hostess, if present, or those at the head table. Place your napkin in your lap when the hostess moves hers. Open full size if it is a lunch napkin, half if it is a large, dinner napkin. Do not refold the napkin at the end of the meal. Leave it unfolded at the right side of the plate.
12. Place the knife and fork at the center of the plate, handles toward the right, when the meal has ended.
13. Wait until the head table, or each person at your table, if at a banquet, is served before beginning to eat.
14. Dip soup away from you. If a bowl must be tipped, tip it away from you.
15. Test hot beverages for "heat or sweet" with one sip from the spoon — one sip only. Then place the spoon on the saucer beside the cup, never on the tablecloth.
16. Refrain from stirring or mashing food on a plate.
17. Put gravy on meat only. If you want gravy on potatoes, or dressing, use your fork to transfer gravy from the meat to these items.

18. Always break bread of any kind at least once before eating. Butter one small bite or one small piece at the time.
19. Bring food to the mouth. Do not lower the head to meet the food.
20. Place a knife, after use, on the other side of the plate, opposite from where you are, with the handle and blade safely on the plate. The handle will point toward the right, slightly toward the person on your right.
21. After cutting meat, put the knife on the other side of the plate, as described above. Transfer the fork to the right hand, and lay the fork down, if in a formal situation, before picking it up again to eat the meat. This casual gesture takes only a few seconds. A relaxed manner is the heart of etiquette and good manners.
22. Grace is said before seating or after seating, before anything is touched on the table. Listen to, and notice, the president or hostess for instructions.
23. Again, never put silver on the table or tablecloth after use.
24. In restaurants, leave a tip of fifteen to twenty percent. Never leave less than twenty-five cents.
25. Again, good manners, and respect and consideration for others precede etiquette if a choice must be made.

Martin Vanbee wrote: "One of the troubles in the world is that we have allowed the Golden Rule to become a bit tarnished."

Ralph Waldo Emerson reminded us: "Life is not so short but that there is always time enough for courtesy."

Chapter 30

Visual Poise

Visual poise is concerned with standing, walking, turning, and sitting correctly and beautifully. Visual refers to what we see or view: poise is graceful movement blended with self-confidence and calm control.

First, let us consider standing correctly.

Standing tall and gracefully begins with good posture. Achieve good posture in one of these two ways:

1. Stand with the back against the wall, heels about three inches from the wall. Shoulders and hips should touch the wall. Lift the chest and pull the stomach muscles inward. Tuck the hips and relax (not drop or droop) the shoulders. No more than the thickness-of-a-hand's space should be between the body and the wall. The spine should be as straight as possible.

2. Stand as tall as possible, head high, chin up, but chin tilted slightly. Raise both hands above the head, as high as possible. Clasp hands above the head. Unclasp and drop hands slowly to one's side. See how straight the body is. Remember: head up, chin slightly tilted, shoulders relaxed, hips tucked and relaxed, tummy in.

Breathe deeply. Think peace and serenity. Relax mentally the face and chest, but do not resume an army-at-ease position.

A beauty contestant had a perfect standing, posture pose, but she was too stiff, too stilted. She lost.

The secret is to practice until one achieves relaxed, good posture.

Standing gracefully involves proper foot placement.

Pretend that you are standing on a stage. The stage is a huge clock. You are facing twelve o'clock.

Move your right foot forward and point it to twelve. Place the left foot behind the right foot and point it toward ten, often referred to as a forty-five degree angle. (The heel of the right foot should be pointing toward the arch of the left foot, about two inches from it.) Turn your body slightly to the left so that viewers see basically at an angle. A full, flat view is often unbecoming.

Walking, turning, and pivoting are important, but easy.

If you are in a situation in which you wish to move forward, begin with the same basic stance described above. Simply step forward slowly with the right foot. If you wish to turn around, shift weight to the toes, with both feet, and turn. This is called a half pivot.

If you wish to do a complete pivot, simply turn on the toes again so that one faces the original direction. (Models often use this in showing clothes from all directions.)

Walking gracefully is an acquired art. (Experts say that each person has an individual style of walking which cannot be changed, but can be improved. In other words, criminologists say that there are three things that cannot be faked completely. They are one's voice, one's handwriting, and one's walk.)

In walking, steps must be short, no more than one's own foot length between steps. Imagine that you are walking on a straight, black line. Do not pigeon-toe in. Walk as straight on the line as possible.

Steps too short make one look older. Steps too long give a masculine look.

Walk lightly. Do not lift the feet too high. The goal is to glide gracefully, not to walk like a soldier.

Practice relaxed breathing as you walk. Let arms swing gracefully and naturally. Be sure to keep them close to the body. Turn palms toward the body. Let hands and fingers relax. Try it. It works.

What does one do with hands when standing?

1. Clasp hands by interlacing fingers, relaxed, in front by letting them drop naturally below the waist. This forms a "V" with the hands and arms, causing one to look smaller and more graceful. (What a woman does with her hands is often the key to her poise and serenity.)
2. Clasp hands behind on one's hips in the same manner.
3. Hold them at one's side, fingers relaxed, with palms turned toward the body.
4. Cross arms in front across the chest, but be sure to let four fingers show with the thumb hidden. Relax fingers. This position can make one look selfish and cold unless it is done correctly.
5. Hold hands in the front, center, at the waist. Turn the palm of the left upward. Lay the right hand in the palm.
6. If you have side pockets, insert the thumb only in the pocket. Let the other four fingers stay outside, relaxed.
7. If you have front pockets, insert all fingers, but let the thumb only stay outside. Keep elbows close to the body.

Hands and eyes are the most expressive parts of a woman's body. Yet, they can be the most distracting. Eyes can express anger, disgust, lack of interest, hate. Improper movement or use of the hands can show signs of nervousness or tension. Keep hands as still as possible. Do not move fingers unnecessarily or "pick at" nails.

Sitting

1. Sit tall. Keep the head erect and the back straight. Never slump.

2. To sit, walk to a chair. Turn on the balls of the feet so that one's back is to the chair.

3. Move close to the chair so that you can feel the chair with the back of the legs. It may be necessary to move one foot slightly forward and the other slightly under the chair to provide balance. Sit slowly, gracefully, and gently. Slide backwards if necessary for comfort. Sit tall.

4. When rising, move to the front of the chair. Push one foot slightly forward, the other backwards toward the chair. Lift hips, keeping the back straight and the head erect. Never push up with the hands.

5. When sitting, never smooth skirts underneath with both hands. Holding one side of the skirt gracefully with one hand is permitted to prevent wrinkling.

6. The most graceful way to sit is to put knees together and feet together. Move the legs slightly, comfortably, to the right side of the chair. Slowly, gently, place the right foot in front of the left. Practice this in front of a full view mirror.

7. Place your hands in your lap, one on top of the other, or put the thumb of the right hand in the palm of the left with fingers to the right hand underneath.

Carrying handbags gracefully

1. Shoulder bags may be supported not only by the shoulder, but also with a graceful clasp of the hand. Also, the strap may be clasped with the thumb, fingers relaxed.

2. Handbags with handles may be carried comfortably near the wrist, palms down. Never turn the palm up when carrying a handbag.

3. An envelope bag is carried close to the body, the hand under the bag with the bag resting in the palm, clasped by the thumb on the outside, the index finger underneath the bag, and the other three fingers on the inside next to the body. Never let the bag extend beyond the elbow. To do so is not safe.

Putting on gloves

1. To don gloves, hold the hand in front near the waist, palm

up. Gently insert the hand. Adjust fingers. Do not hold the glove downward and plunge hand in.

2. To remove gloves, hold the hand in front near the waist. Remove the glove by working gently with the opposite hand, beginning with the palm and working with the fingers. For a more attractive donning or removing, keep palms up as much as possible.

Getting into a car

1. To get into a car from the passenger's side, or the driver's side, stand beside the car, facing the front of the car. Lower yourself into the car, hips in first. When seated, follow by lifting feet and legs together into the car.

2. To get out of a car, slip to the side of the seat next to the door. Swing feet out together. When feet are on the earth, lift the body to a standing position.

Making introductions

1. Introductions confuse us. Learn one or two correct ways and use them.

2. Say: "May I introduce?" or "May I present?" Also, "This is John" is acceptable.

3. Say an older person's name before saying a younger. Mrs. Jones, may I present Sue Smith? Mr. Smith, this is Jack Tedder.

4. Say a woman's name before saying a man's. Miss Jones, may I present Jack Jones?

5. Say a married woman's name before a single woman. Mrs. Smith, this is Miss Kigle.

6. Acknowledge introductions with a simple "How do you do?"

    A gracious person can add: "Mrs. Jones is a former student of mine," or an appropriate statement for continuing conversation purposes.

Putting on a coat and taking off a coat

1. Putting on a coat involves four steps:

A. Hold the coat by the collar in the right hand in front of you, lining facing you.
B. Insert the left arm in the left sleeve.
C. Slide the right arm into the right sleeve.
D. Adjust and button or tie.

Move graciously, gracefully, and slowly. Do all things with a touch of elegance.

2. Taking off a coat or removing a coat involves four steps:

A. Grasp lightly the front lapels with each hand to help the coat slide off the shoulders slightly.
B. Reach back with both hands.
C. Catch and hold both sleeves with the left hand as you bring both hands to the front.
D. Catch both sleeves with the right hand, slide left arm out, and place the neatly-folded coat over the arm.

Visual poise is synonymous with that special touch of elegance which is so much a part of the beautiful, caring woman.

Chapter 31

Non-Verbal Communication

Not all communication is spoken or written. The saying, "Action speaks louder than words" is true. Experts say that over fifty percent of what we communicate is nonverbal. This is frightening.

You see, we thought that we could be careful what we say and all would be all right.

Not so. We say much about ourselves by the way we sit, walk, or stand. We also communicate with our dress, appearance, attitude, facial expressions, and behavior.

Seeing is as important in communication as hearing. Have you ever turned down the sound on the television to answer the phone — and continued to watch the program with understanding?

Have you ever been in an adjoining room listening to a program on a television in another room, only to re-enter the room where the television is and ask, "What is happening?"

Non-verbal communication can be very misleading. Watch the characters on television, especially those who are foils. Notice how much action and expression are used to reveal character and personality.

A woman who seemed very proud was described by her peers as having an inferiority complex. A woman who laughed very much was known to be very insecure and afraid.

Ann Landers wrote:

> "Laughter is an intensely personal thing. Some people chuckle, others cackle or hoot, and others only smile. The phony laugh seldom passes for the real thing. I will always remember the comment of a Chinese friend. He said, 'Many Americans must be very unhappy. They laugh so much.' "[1]

During the Watergate hearings, viewers were challenged to watch the eyes for evidence of deceit or dishonesty. Have you ever seen the voiceograms in papers showing that things are not always as they seem? The voice and the eyes "give us away." Truth, genuineness, and sincerity never fail, in verbal or non-verbal communication.

Many marriages fail, we are told, because of lack of communication. Though words may not be spoken, many non-verbal communications are expressed as long as people attempt to live together. Actions, movements, and expressions show disgust, disdainment, rejection, and even hatred. People who go to marriage counselors complain that words not spoken are far more cruel than words expressed. How tragic — when there is so much love and beauty in the world — so many beautiful things not said or thought until it is too late.

Chapter 32

Using Time Wisely

B enjamin Franklin once asked: "Dost thou love
life?" After waiting for a moment for an answer,
he replied: "Then do not squander time, for that is
the stuff that life is made of."

So often we wonder, "How does a certain person
seem to accomplish so much?"

Maybe we should just let that remain a rhetorical
question because the ability of certain people and their
success in accomplishing much will always remain a
mystery.

Yet, somewhere we may find an answer, an explanation, if we seek diligently.

First, many people work while the rest of the world
sleeps or plays or vacations. The LADDER OF SAINT
AUGUSTINE seems to say it best:

> "The heights of great men reached and kept
>   Were not attained by sudden flight,
>   But, they, while their companions slept
>   Were toiling upward in the night."

Second, there are ways that one can "control" time.

One of the major complaints of the world is "I don't have time to do that."

The essence of time exists, to a great extent, in the mind. One is not being sacrilegious when one says that one can almost control time, especially as it relates to one's own life.

Try this. If you live ten miles from the nearest town, plan a one-hour venture from your home into town to do several errands, and to park — in sixty minutes.

On paper, write:

1. Buy a loaf of bread at the grocery store
2. Buy stamps and mail letter
3. Leave the hymnals at the church
4. Get check cashed
5. Pick up prescription at the drug store
6. Park the car

Dress. Get everything in order. Starting at a timed moment, drive into town, calmly, quietly, thoughtfully, with the list at one's side. Do not use time to talk or to shop for items not on the list. Do all this in one hour. You may have minutes "left over." Don't doubt that this can be done until you have tried it.

Third, use time when you are alone to accomplish miracles.

Carl Sandburg wrote: "Shakespeare, da Vinci, Franklin, and Lincoln never saw a movie, heard a radio, or looked at television. They had loneliness and knew what to do with it. They were not afraid of being lonely because they knew that was when the creative mood in them would work."

When the family or friends or associates are away, work, work, work. Think, think, think. Plan, plan, plan. Do, do, do!

Fourth, life is like a piano: what you get out of it depends on how you play it. Success and achievement require hard work, sacrifice, self-discipline, and beyond-the-ordinary effort. Again, it often means working while the rest of the world sleeps.

Fifth, make a list. This is an age-old recommendation, but it works like magic. Just make a list of things that you must do and mark them off as you do them. In some inexplicable way, this saves time. It also saves the headache of remembering.

If I could start my life again, I would keep a diary or a list or an account or a journal of all the events of my life, day by day — people, places, events, telephone numbers, addresses, thoughts, feelings, actions, reactions. This would have saved me much time and would have given me much joy in reminiscing.

Sixth, there is a very "touchy" use of time that must be mentioned. A very old friend who had a very talkative, long-visiting neighbor gave this advice: "Don't allow people to 'use up' your life."

People are the ultimate of God's creation. They are all-important. But there are those who seem to have more time to use in using the time of others. One must be very discreet. A friend in need is the most important thought of the moment or time, but long visits, long telephone conversations, and other events which take much time must be eliminated beyond reason unless one chooses to prolong. Be simple, sincere, and courteous, but "depart from these," if you wish, if you choose, if you must. They "use up" one's life.

Seventh, in using time, do not compare your accomplishments with others. Some of the things that people do are more visible to the human eye than others. If I write a book, it may be seen or read, but if you say a prayer, it may bring events that will change the world without anyone's ever knowing.

Eighth, "Time will pass. Will you?" This was a quotation that hung beneath a classroom clock. It provided food for thought to many students.

We look at our clocks or watches many times each day at work, at school, or wherever we are. We often wonder why time does not pass more quickly or why time passes so quickly. Yet, the all-important question is this: "Will we pass the test of time?"

This thought brings us to the sacred. Let us begin with this lovely Irish prayer:

"Take time to work: it is the price of success.
Take time to think: it is the source of power.
Take time to play: it is the secret of perpetual youth.
Take time to read: it is the foundation of wisdom.
Take time to be friendly: it is the road to happiness.
Take time to love and be loved: it is the privilege of the gods.
Take time to share: life is too short to be selfish.
Take time to laugh: Laughter is the music of the soul."

The most beautiful thoughts concerning time are found in Ecclesiastes 3:1-8:

"To every thing there is a season, and a time to every purpose under heaven:

A time to be born and a time to die; a time to plant and a time to pluck up that which is planted;

A time to kill and a time to heal; a time to break down and a time to build up;

A time to weep and a time to laugh; a time to mourn, and a time to dance;

A time to cast away stones, and a time to gather stones together; a time to embrace, and a time to refrain from embracing;

A time to get, and a time to lose; a time to keep, and a time to cast away;

A time to rend, and a time to sew; a time to keep silence, and a time to speak;

A time to love, and a time to hate; a time of war, and a time of peace.

The HOLY BIBLE, King James Version

Chapter 33

Word Pronunciations and Practical Grammar

To realize the profound effect that the voice has on beauty is a paradox: It is both frightening and exhilarating.

The sound of the voice — the intonation, the tone, the pronunciation, the enunciation — can make the loveliest person unattractive or the most homely person lovely.

As has been mentioned earlier in this book, artificiality and superficiality in speech are detestable. The human voice is a gem that needs only to be polished and perfected to its purest natural state. Again, any voice affectations are deplorable.

The voice must be well-modulated, clear, and sincere — the instrument through which pure, perfect words and thoughts flow. This does not mean that we must be perfect: we cannot be until eternity. This does not mean that we must be so afraid to speak that we become unnatural because we are so conscious of what we say, so aware!

Again, the goal is to quieten our lives and our voices,

to practice deep breathing, and to learn a few basic rules of correct speech so that we shall feel secure and unafraid.

Let us consider pronunciation first. It is difficult to give exact, synonymous sounds. Check diacritical marks in a good dictionary if the following explanations are not clear.

1. Let us begin with a difficult group. Say nature, temperature, furniture, literature. The latter three have the same sound as nature. The preferred pronunciation is *chur*, not *ture*. Many say *ture* and emphasize it. *Chur* is preferred and is not emphasized. (There are other possible pronunciations of *literature,* probably the most overbearingly mispronounced, "mis-emphasized" word in the field of education.) Again, say "nature, temperature, furniture, and literature," and make them rhyme: you will come out honorably.
2. The "t" in *often* is not pronounced. Say "off-en."
3. The word *coffee* does not rhyme with "law." Try the sound of "co" in "cop."
4. The word *water* does not include the sound of "r." Say "Wah-ter."
5. The word *again* is not pronounced "ah-gain." Try "ah-gan" as if one is saying the "an" in "an egg." Try again and say "an" for the final syllable. Do not say "an" with a "flat" sound. Say "an" at the tip of the tongue and the front of the mouth and it will come out right.
6. The word *once* must not include the sound of "t."
7. *Where* rhymes with "air."
8. *There* rhymes with "air." But be sure to say the word *air* correctly, at the front of the mouth, not at the back of the mouth or in the throat.
9. *Hair* and *air* do not have the same sound as "Harold," unless "Harold" is also sounded at the front of the mouth.
10. Say *every* day, not "ever" day.
11. Say *was*, not "wuz."
12. For *oil, boil, toil, spoil, soil* one does not say "ol" or

"bol" or "tol." Try "oy-yul," "boy-yul," "toy-yul." We say these words as we do many others — with too much "flat" sound. Listen to a good television commentator to see how he or she says *oil*.

13. *Dormitory* is not "domitory." The word has an "r." Sound the "r."

14. *Secretary* is not "sek-ku-tary." Sound the "cre" as in "creed," without the "ed," of course. In other words, sound "cre."

15. *Mrs.* is not "miseries." A married woman is not necessarily miserable, so do not call her a "miseries." The sound is "Miz-z." This is "Miz-z" (Mrs.) Jones.

16. The sound of *Misses* is "Miss-es," with the sound of "s." The two Misses Clarks will perform.

17. *Ought* rhymes with bought, thought, sought, and fought. It is not pronounced as "ort."

18. Put the "t" on east and west.

Watch the overuse or incorrect use of *of, up,* and *on*:

1. inside of — omit the of
2. outside of — omit the of
3. later on — omit the on
4. added on — omit the on
5. burned up — omit the up
6. over with — omit the with

We are concerned about ending sentences with prepositions. The problem usually involves unnecessary prepositions such as those above. For example, in the sentence, "Where did you put it at?" the word *at* is superfluous or unnecessary. But "What are you looking at?" is a good sentence with no superfluous "at." In conversation, the preceding sentence is more effective than "At what are you looking?" Both sentences are correct.

My favorite example of the fanaticism of not ending a

sentence with a preposition is illustrated by the statement that Sir Winston Churchill made during the critical days of World War II. In a famous speech, he said, "That is something that England will not put up with!"

Immediately, the critics condemned him for ending a sentence with a preposition.

His quick reply was: "The next time I want to impress the enemy I will say, 'That is something up with which England will not put!'"

1. threw, not throwed
2. grew, not growed
3. first, not firstly
4. second, not secondly
5. third, not thirdly
6. exactly, not just exactly

We are often afraid to use the words *sung* and *rung*. These words are "very correct." They are the past participles: ring, rang, rung, and sing, sang, sung. Do not use them alone as verbs. Use them with had, has, have, is, are, was, or were in front of them. If they are used as "pure participles," however, they may be used alone as "The song, sung in unison, was beautiful." In the preceding sentence, as was stated, *sung* is not a verb, but a verbal, a participle. Again, "He sung a song," is incorrect. One must say "He sang a song," or "He has sung a song."

The following are correct because they are accepted as correct with no grammatical explanation:

1. I shall try *to* go (not *try and*).
2. He lives *away* up the hill, (not *way up*).
3. He lives *a long way* from here, (not *a long ways*).

Avoid the use of muchly for *much*, enthused for *en-*

thusiastic, gent for *gentleman,* heartrendering for *heartrending,* unbeknowst for *unknown,* over with (another unnecessary preposition) for *over.*

Pronounce the "h" in *humble,* but do not pronounce the "h" in *prohibition.*

Words have strong connotations or suggested meanings:

1. Casket, not coffin
2. Took his life, not committed suicide
3. Passed away, not died
4. Deceased, for dead
5. Mental hospital or mental institution, or asylum for the insane, not insane asylum
6. Shampooed hair, instead of washed hair
7. Showered, rather than took a bath or bathed

Overuse of the expressions *a lot, lots, very, O.K.,* and *okay* should be watched.

If I had to select two pet peeves, these would be the overuse of "you know," and the use of "kids" for children or young people.

To hear young people of school age, kindergarten through twelve, referred to as "kids" is very disturbing. But to hear a college or university coach refer to members of his or her team as "kids" is even more upsetting.

Consider the following:

1. Use *rear* for "raised" in referring to rearing children.
2. Use *remember* instead of "recollect."
3. Say *friend* rather than "personal friend."
4. Say "over" rather than "over with."
5. Avoid the expression *point blank.*
6. Use the expression *each other* to refer to two, as "The twins helped each other," and *one another* to refer to more than two, as "The members of the family helped one another."

7. Watch the incorrect use of *same* when a word such as *it* should be used. For example, avoid: "They bought the meat and ate same." Or "I received the letter and I am answering same."
8. Avoid saying "awfully tired" or "terribly tired." These are incorrect uses of awful and terrible.
9. Do not confuse *less* and *fewer*. *Fewer* refers to number; *less* to amount. (fewer mistakes, less time).
10. Use *empty* with such words as bottles, *vacant* with buildings.
11. Avoid the use of such expressions as "fantastic," "at this point in time," "frame of reference," "you can say that again," "due to the fact," "right!" and "really?"

One of the most beautiful polishes to the English language is the use of the possessive case (my, your, his, her its, our, your, their) before an *ing* word that is a gerund.

> He had not heard of my going (not me going).
> your going (not you going).
> his going (not him going).
> our going (not us going).
> their going (not them going).

Many other much-used words require the possessive as "ing" forms of the gerund: my telling, my asking, my finding, my showing and hundreds of others.

Another "polish" is the use of *really* instead of *real* before a predicate adjective. Usually, *really* is correct if *very* is appropriate.

> Say, "I am really tired," not real tired. One could say "very tired," so the word *really* may be substituted. Try "really pleased," "really concerned," and others.

A professor told a class of prospective teachers that one of the strongest words to add to their vocabulary was *let's*. Another superb idea is "Maybe it would be better to consider . . ." Too, pad a negative with a polite, sincere positive: "I should really like to attend, but. . . ."

Pronouns give us more trouble than any other element in speaking. The forms I, you, he, she, we, you, and they are used as subjects and also as what we call predicate nominatives which come after or follow the words is, are, was, were, am, be, been. This is why we say "This is she," rather than "This is her."

The pronouns me, you, him, her, us, you, and them are objects. He saw me. He told us. Simple? Yes. But the compounds trouble us.

"Mary and I are going" (subject) but "She told Mary and me" (object). To check these, omit half of the compound. "She told me," sounds natural and correct — and it is.

An expression that causes much pain and uncertainty is "I feel bad." We want to say "I feel badly" because we think we have or need an adverb to answer the question "feel how?" Not so. The reason: The words *seem* or *seems, appear* or *appears, look* or *looks, taste* or *tastes, feel* or *feels, smell* or *smells,* and *sounds* or *sound* are followed by adjectives, not adverbs.

> He seems happy, not happily.
> He looks happy, not happily.
> The cake tastes sweet, not sweetly.
> He feels bad, not badly.
> The milk tastes sour, not sourly.
> The heart sounds good, not well.
>
> (Good, better, best are adjectives. Well, better, best are adverbs.)

One must watch these. Sometimes, though rarely,

one will find an example when meaning makes a difference. For example, one could need to say to a doctor: "Since I injured my hand, I feel badly with these fingers. I seem to have no sense of touch." Or one says, "The horn sounds too loud. Could you adjust it for me?" Yet, it may be necessary to say. "The horn sounded loudly through the woodlands when the hunter blew it."

The correct pronunciation of words is a problem. Let us always be sure to say this all-important word correctly: America! Say "Ah-mer-ree-kah" with four syllables, not "Ah-mer-cah."

If one lives in North Carolina or South Carolina, or needs to say the names of these, say "Care-oh-line-ah," with four syllables, not "Care-line-ah."

Another most-often-mispronounced word that all of us use is mischievous. It is pronounced "miss-chi-vus" with the emphais on the "miss" part, not "miss-*cheeve*-e-us," as most of us say. If we pronounce it incorrectly, we shall surely spell it incorrectly.

There is a world of words that we mispronounce by putting the emphasis on the wrong syllable. Here are a few. The syllable that is capitalized is the one emphasized: *PREF*erable, *VE*hicle, *DIS*cipline, *EX*quisite, *VE*hement, *AM*nesty, *LAM*entable, in*COM*parable, *COM*parable, ir*REP*arable, in*DIC*ative, advan*TAG*eous, *SES*ame, as*PIR*ant, *IN*dustry, *AN*cestor, *IN*famous, *HOS*pitable, *DEF*icit, i*DE*a, *IN*teresting, *THE*atre, and *MIS*chievous.

Others include e*PIT*ome, *IM*potent, the*SAU*rus, *IN*fluence, a*BYSS*, ver*BOSE*, su*PER*fluous, *POST*humous, *IM*petus, fi*NA*le, inde*FAT*igable, *BAR*barous, bar*BAR*ic, *MEM*orable, in*TER*, *PAS*toral, ma*NI*acal, in*TER*ment, am*BIG*uous, un*PREC*edented, re*CON*-naissance, *DEP*rivation, *AU*topsy, *SI*ren, *SPIG*ot.

The following give us trouble also:

route (root), kiln (kill), thresh (not thrash), seance (SAYans), real (not reel), your (rhymes with moor, tour), wan (rhymes with don, con), with (sound the th), skein (skane), respite (RESpit), poor (rhymes with moor, tour), yacht (yot), via (rhymes with higher), gubernatorial (guber, not goober), greasy (not greazy), apropos (apropo), fungi (funjeye), guano (gwano), sol-der (the 1 is silent), resin (REZin, not RAWsin), rinse (not wrench), roof, coop, root, and hoof (all four with long oo as in food), height (hite), quantity (sound the t), government (sound the n), recognize (sound the g), conspicuous (sound the u, uous), fact (sound the t), in-sect (sound the t), bronchial (brong ki al), diphtheria (dif), niche (nitch), wish (not wush), extra (ah), pretty (say pritty), draught (draft), bestial (bestyal), clique (kleek), mauve (rhymes with rove), liaison (leeaZON), debris (dayBREE), corps (core), population (sound the u), strength (not strenth), forehead (FARed), apologize (sound the final o), pamphlet (pamflet), nude (newd, not nood), salmon (samun), American (kan, not kun), chasm (kasm), wrestle (not rassle), elm (not ellum), culinary (kew, not kul), and inch (not eench). Also, remember athlete (ath lete) and athletics (ath letics) with no center "e" sounded.

Certain words such as laissez faire (lassy FAIR), coup d'etat (KOO day TA) or esprit de corps (esPRE de KOR) may cause us concern. Also, alumnus (aLUM-nus), alumni (aLUMnye), alumna (aLUMna), and alumnae (aLUMnee).

If one is in doubt concerning pronunciation, one can

readily consult a dictionary. Diacritical marks and pronunciation guides can always lead to perfection.

Chapter 34

Exercise

This could appropriately be called "The Age of Exercise," for we are involved in exercise and jogging emphasis. Almost every monthly magazine concerned with health and beauty has an article on this subject.

The American Heart Association, the Alliance for Health, Physical Education, Recreation, and Dance, the American College of Sports Medicine, and the President's Council on Physical Fitness and Sports, and other leading organizations have encouraged and supported the principle that our society should become more physically active. However, exercise must not be thought of as a cure-all in rehabilitation or preventive medicine, but as one of the elements of a healthier, happier lifestyle.

There is convincing evidence that regular exercise, combined with proper diet, relaxation, and wise management of stress, contribute to less morbidity and mortality as well as to better health and more efficient performance.

Regular exercise, like dieting, requires discipline. Discipline requires doing what must be done at the time that it should be done. Almost half of the population of the United States gives up sports after finishing high school, according to the President's Council for Physical Fitness and Sports. Of 45 million Americans over the age of 55, estimates are that only about 30 percent exercise.

Exercising could truthfully be called "medicising" because exercise is good "medicine."

The heart is the powerhouse of the body. If the heart is normal, it will beat approximately 100,000 times per day, a million times every ten days, and between 36 and 38 million times every year. Each day the heart pumps from five to ten tons of blood.

One way to improve the heart and keep the blood moving, with its lubricating, cleansing, and reviving action is through a regular jogging, walking, exercising program.

Exercise gives one a sense of well-being, relieves tension, and makes one feel good. Mental, emotional, and spiritual benefits have been proved. Muscles become stronger, and respiration is improved. Try it! It works!

Psychiatrists at the University of Wisconsin found that exercise definitely helps patients suffering from moderate depression. Dr. John Greist found that patients who did not respond to antidepressant drugs responded to exercise such as walking or running for thirty minutes three or four times each week.

Exercise improves breathing. Good breathing techniques can help control, and even cure, headaches, depression, dizziness, and insomnia. Deep breathing can help eliminate fatigue and tension.

The President's Council on Physical Fitness has prepared a 64-page booklet, "Adult Physical Fitness," an illustrated guide for men and women who want to undertake a fitness program. It is available for seventy cents from the Consumer Information Center, Department 088F, Pueblo, Colorado 81009.

If one gets plenty of rest and eats well, but becomes exhausted by four o'clock in the afternoon, government experts say that gradual deterioration of the body because of the lack of physical exercise could be the cause. Chronic fatigue ranks as one of the most common complaints today.

Exercising could readily be called "movasizing" because it involves movement, and it can help to move the size of clothing that one wears. All movement is exercise, but one must go beyond the everyday, life-demanding efforts to get the maximum benefits of exercise.

Americans spend billions of dollars each year on makeup, hair dyes, face lifts, and fine clothes — all trying to make themselves feel better. Too often we forget that the best things in life are free. Exercise is a good example.

Never underestimate the value of the ever-popular calisthenics which all of us recall from grammar school. Touching toes, arm circles, "squat-ups-and downs," side bends, arm swings, and neck rounds all added to our youthful strength.

The best exercise book that I have found is the official ROYAL CANADIAN AIR FORCE EXERCISE PLANS FOR PHYSICAL FITNESS, revised U.S. edition, with the XBX plan for women and the 5BX plan for men. Be sure to get the exact title listed above, approximately 8½ by 5½ inches. There is a similar title that is not so good. The book sells for about $3.00.

Bowling, brisk walking, swimming, jumping rope, tennis, bicycling, golf, jogging, jumping on a trampoline-type mat, weight-lifting, volleyball, and other forms of exercise should be considered. Choice will vary according to environment, lifestyle, age, and time available.

Country living has many advantages, one of which is the freedom to walk or jog. If you are fortunate to have this advantage, measure, by car, if you wish, a certain distance. In this way, you will know how far you are walking. Because no one is watching, be free, be creative with your walking. Take giant steps, feeling muscles moving. Take short, prancing steps, like a majorette, or walk as "prissy" as you can, throwing hips to each side as far as possible, as you walk. Do arm circles. Breathe deeply. Pull in the tummy as far as possible and hold. Again, be creative. You will be surprised how many muscles you can move or feel.

Slow running or jogging uses about the same number of calories per mile as ordinary walking. An average-size person of 145 pounds will use about 60 calories per mile more than he or she would use if sitting for the same length of time. One will use fewer calories if he weighs less than 145; more, if he weighs more than 145.

If one walks two miles each day, that is 120 calories burned or used, 840 per week, and 3360 per month. A pound of fat contains about 3500 calories. So, if one walked two miles each day, one could lose 12 pounds per year if one also ate sensibly.

When exercising inside, if one wears leotards, or

clothing with short sleeves, or shorts, it is interesting to exercise in front of a mirror. This helps one to see many of the muscles and skin areas that are actually benefiting. For example, if one extends the arms for circling or does back-kicking or side-kicking with the legs, one can easily observe fat, and movement of that fat, when exercising before a mirror.

The slant board (described in chapter 26) is the best device I have found for doing calisthenics in a lying position. The board allows all kinds of leg lifts, push-ups, bicycling, scissoring — all — without excess strain. Try it! It works!

A WORD OF CAUTION

Exercise and jogging must be purely motivated and perfectly controlled. Excess and obsessions are out! Improved health, more zest, energy, and vitality, better breathing and greater strength are the goals. Any irrational responses to subconscious anxieties such as the fountain-of-youth-stay-younger-longer-never-die theories will perhaps prove worthless. Even though exercising brings long-range benefits, the chief joys should be a part of now.

The secret of good health is to get in touch with one's body, to listen to its messages, and to interpret its sensations, altering our lifestyle whether it involves nutrition, exercise, rest, sleep, or any other change.

If we will listen, our body will speak to us. Responding will not only lead to preventive medicine, but also to better health.

Chapter 35

Dieting: Heaps of Hints to Help

Much pain comes to us from (1) what does into our mouths and (2) what comes from our mouths. The former concerns eating, the latter, speaking. This chapter is concerned with food and diet. Other chapters consider speech.

We cannot change many things in life: our nationality, race, innate talents or lack of them, our height, or the color of our eyes.

However, obesity, or being overweight, a problem that plagues over 80 million Americans, is one thing that we can do something about if we choose, for it is said that overeating is a learned habit. But that is not all bad. Habits can be broken: habits can be un-learned.

The formulas and methods are very simple. In fact, losing weight is so easy that people do not believe what they read about it. If losing weight cost a fortune, or called for a long journey to a strange place, or required complicated procedures, all the world, or much of it, would travel, even flock, in that direction.

As has been suggested, the word should be "do-it"

instead of diet — because that is what it amounts to — doing it. Can you imagine going around saying, "I'm on a "do-it." Yet, if any diet is successful, that is what a diet is all about — doing it.

Doing what?

1. First, we go back to the philosophy of this book — simplicity. We eliminate or decrease the foods we now eat — fats, sweets, and starches, especially. Imagine how that would cut one's grocery bill.
2. We live one day at a time, and we diet one day at a time. Anything can be endured for a day.
3. Someone has said, "The trick is to stick."
4. Eat what is good for you, not what is good to you, especially if the two are not the same. In other words, eat what you need, not what you want. The saying, "Eat to live, not live to eat," is always good advice.
5. For good health and good nutrition, eat a little of everything and not too much of anything.
6. Say to yourself, "I have eaten enough. I may feel hungry, but I am not going to starve. I have 'fed myself and fed myself well.' I may think I am going to 'faint and fall out,' but I really am not. I shall survive if I endure — and I will!"
7. Shirley Bright Boody, registered dietician of Copley News Service wrote: "A lot of people have self-image problems after losing so much weight . . . There are many reasons why some people are more comfortable when they are fat. Some may view fat as a sort of protection. Others use it to avoid sexual encounters, or to escape certain job or home activities.

   "Each night before you go to bed, visualize yourself as slender, and take pride in how you look. Enjoy and delight in every pound lost, knowing that each one is contributing to a healthier you."[1]

Again, over 80 million Americans are overweight. A USDA report released on July 5, 1981, stated that one in every five people in the United States is on a diet. In a recent USDA survey, 61 percent of the households sampled included at least one person who had tried to lose weight in the past year.

Over 31 diseases are directly associated with obesity. Do we want to be thin, strong, and healthy, or do we want to be overweight and possibly become ill? Doctors point out that the chief concern is not always the fat that shows on the outside, but the fat that may have accumulated on the inside around vital organs.

Over $80 million is spent annually on weight reduction in America. Can we not find a more sensible way of eating and save a great deal of money for happy things?

Food allergies, nutritional unbalance, and excess cause behavioral disturbances and lead to violent behavior, depression, and serious physical and emotional illness. Need we to say more?

Dieting and being overweight are subjects "closest to my heart." When I was a child, a little girl was supposed to look like Shirley Temple. I was far from that image! My hair was straight, I was not nearly so intelligent as Shirley Temple, and I was overweight.

When I graduated from high school, I weighed about twenty or twenty-five pounds more than the charts recommended.

As I write this, I am attending Diet Workshop, one and one-half pounds from the recommended goal.

So, for over twenty-five years, losing weight has been an obsession, a continuing, ever-present obsession to me. Because, so far as I know, I have not had health problems related to my obesity, I suppose it must be a matter of vanity, even though being always "too heavy on one's feet" is a constant physical discomfort.

With so many personal concerns, as well as an

awareness of world problems, especially those related to starvation and hunger, one often gets a feeling of guilt from being concerned about weight, especially if one needs to lose only ten or fifteen pounds — for vanity, more than health reasons.

Nevertheless, vanity takes its toll.

Maybe it is a matter of good stewardship of one's body. Maybe it is remembering that ". . . ye are the temple of God, and that the Spirit of God dwelleth in you" (I Corinthians 3:16).

Consider the following:

1. Before dieting, see a doctor, especially if one has more than ten pounds to lose. A person is considered obese when that person has at least twenty excessive pounds.
2. Eat three meals each day. For snacks, choose fruits such as apples, bananas, or oranges, or fresh vegetables that can be eaten raw. The word *diet* has the word *die* in it. Our appetite, hunger, or craving for rich, high calorie food must die — and they will if we cultivate our tastes long enough to create a change.
3. Use salt sparingly, if at all.
4. Buy an inexpensive, small calorie counter. Choose low-calorie foods.
5. Avoid sweets, pastries, cookies, cakes, cream, fats, sauces, gravies, fried foods, fat and fat meat, and colas that are non-dietetic.
6. Increase activities and exercise.
7. Eat meat in moderation (3 ounces of red meat per day or 4-6 ounces of white meat such as fish, poultry, or veal).
8. Learn to like low calorie, low fat foods such as cottage cheese, which is high in protein.
9. Plan your diet around available foods and recipes. Only in this way will the diet become a lifetime plan.
10. If the food we eat provides more energy (calories) than we need, the extra energy (calories) will be stored as fat. If the foods we eat provide less energy than is needed, the

body will use fat that is stored.

11. Each person burns about one calorie each minute, regardless of activity. Therefore, we burn 60 calories each hour, simply by living. This totals 1440 per day.
12. Much of the weight that people lose from fad diets is water weight. This weight quickly returns.
13. An "empty calorie" is a phrase used to indicate that a food substance contains calories but no important vitamins and minerals. Alcohol is an example.
14. Items labeled "low calorie" must contain no more than 40 calories per serving, and no more than 0.4 calories per gram. There are 28.5 grams in an ounce.
15. To be labeled "reduced calorie," a food must be at least one-third lower in calories than a similar food which has not been reduced.
16. Foods labeled "low calorie" and "reduced calorie" must meet Federal standards. Foods must not be nutritionally inferior to foods to which they are compared.
17. Water is a good aid in combating hunger. Try it. It works.
18. Vitamins are not pep pills and have no calorie or energy value of their own.
19. Eliminate "pure" sugar. Bodies do not require sugar, as such. We get enough sugar from nutritious foods such as milk and grains, fruits and vegetables.
20. Researchers have determined that environment has a greater influence on obesity than heredity.
21. Some obesity is caused by glandular imbalance or other physical problems. A doctor is needed to assist if one has trouble losing weight after dedicated effort.
22. Many excellent diet books and pamphlets are available, many of which are free, from the U.S. Department of Agriculture and/or The U.S. Government Printing Office, Washington, D.C. One of these that is superior is DIETARY GOALS FOR THE UNITED STATES, prepared by the staff of the Select Committee on Nutrition and Human Needs, United States Senate. Order from the U.S. Printing Office, Washington, D.C., of course.
23. A challenge to the overeater is to find the cause for overeating and to do something about it.

The Heart of the Dieting Matter

1. A pound of fat contains about 3500 calories. It takes about 1400 calories per day for the body to carry on normal functions such as heartbeats, digestion, and breathing.

    Suppose that you are a person who burns 600 calories each day in movement and activities. That means that you can use 2000 calories per day.

    Consider, for example, that you eat food containing 3500 calories. You will have eaten 1500 extra calories, and thus, you will gain weight.

2. To lose a pound of body fat a week, one needs to have a calorie deficit of about 3500 calories. If one leaves off 500 calories each day, he should lose a pound each week unless he is eating exorbitant amounts of food.

    For example, if you determine that you are eating food containing 2000 calories, and that you need to lose weight, simply cut your calories by 500 per day, eat only 1500, and you will lose one pound per week.

    Use a calorie counter to help you determine the calories in your food.

3. Again, to lose one pound, a person must consume 3500 fewer calories than the body needs or burns. In other words, to lose weight, "leave off" food, or find ways to "burn it up" or use its energy.

4. Learn to omit foods that contain calories, specifically fat. These are 9 calories per gram of fat and only 4 calories per gram of carbohydrates or protein.

5. No matter how well-balanced the diet, never cut daily calorie intake to below 1000 calories.

6. Do not try to trick nature by trying to lose weight too rapidly. The body has a protective system that will fight your efforts in time of starvation attempts or illness. One can lose water rapidly, and risk dehydration, but losing fat requires a slow, patient process.

7. The word DIET comes from the Greek word meaning "a manner of living." Remember, that for most of us, dieting and calorie-counting must become a way of life if we are to lose weight successfully and keep it off permanently.

Consider these possible reasons for overeating: physical, such as those related to the thyroid, other glands, or chemistry of the body; fatigue; boredom; habit; nervous tension; lack of knowledge concerning calories; influence of younger years; lack of knowledge concerning nutrition; lifestyle; inherent tastes — possibly acquired; and pleasure.

Those persons now in their seventies were parents during the Great Depression. Persons in the fifty-year-old group were born during the Great Depression. Though many boast that "we did not have much, but we always had enough to eat," those persons may have been exaggerating. Many ate much, if food was available, seeking a feeling of security or freedom from hunger. Even children ate many carbohydrates and fats until they felt "full." Therefore, a feeling of fullness became a necessary sensation before leaving the table.

It takes about twenty minutes for food to reach the stomach to give a feeling of satisfaction. If one eats heartily for twenty minutes, too much food is consumed. That is why eating slowly is highly recommended. Eat longer, but eat less.

Psychologists suggest that size and weight are to some people a symbol of power. "The Big Mama" title or "Big Daddy" image are more meaningful than some admit. Often, it is a subconscious, even unconscious, kind of thing.

One woman of middle age said that she did not want to be remembered as the largest woman who had lived in her village. "I thought there was much more honor in being remembered for having the courage to lose excessive weight," she beamed.

Insecure husbands are afraid for their wives to lose

weight. Insecure wives are afraid for their husbands to lose weight. The simple truth of these two statements requires no further explanation.

Some persons have a persecution complex. They seem to hate themselves. Their self-concepts are low: they really want to be overweight.

Obesity basically means "eating oneself fat." The challenge is to find the underlying cause and then find a good diet to correct the problem. Health is first: appearance is second.

An old English proverb states: "Gluttony slays more than the sword," and in the early eighteenth century, Thomas Fuller wrote: "More die by food than by famine."

Where are we — and why are we there?

Maybe we cannot answer. But we can act. We can find a good diet and "do-it."

In an effort to show that "calories do count," I searched diligently for comparative charts and menus to show how addition of certain ingredients or methods of preparation changed caloric content. Finally, in the United States Department of Agriculture's bulletin, FOOD: A PUBLICATION ON FOOD AND NUTRITION (Home and Garden Bulletin Number 228), I found the perfect answer on page 11 in a section entitled "Calorie Countdown." Though this bulletin, like others by USDA, is in the public domain, Robert J. Anzelmo, Acting Assistant Head, Publishing Center, USDA, Washington, D.C. 20250, graciously consented to the use of this excellent material.

CALORIE COUNTDOWN
(Calorie values are shown in parentheses.)

Fruit and Vegetable Group

Lower	In-Between	Higher
1 cup raw vegetable salad without dressing (40)[1]	¾ cup raw vegetable salad with 1 tablespoon French dressing (95)	½ cup potato salad (125)
½ cup cooked cabbage (15)	½ cup coleslaw (60)	2 rolls stuffed cabbage (260)
1 medium baked potato (95)	⅔ cup mashed potatoes prepared with milk and butter (125)	½ cup hashed brown potatoes (170)
1 medium raw apple (80)	1 sweetened baked apple (160)	⅛ of 9-inch apple pie (300)
½ cup fresh citrus sections (40)	½ cup jellied citrus salad (120)	½ cup lemon pudding (145)
½ cup cooked green beans (15)	½ cup stir-fried green beans (35)	½ cup green bean-mushroom casserole (70)
½ cup diced fresh pineapple (40)	½ cup canned pineapple chunks in natural juice (70)	½ cup canned pineapple chunks in heavy sirup (95)

Bread and Cereal Group

Lower	In-Between	Higher

1 cup plain corn flakes (95)	1 cup sugar-coated cornflakes (155)	½ cup crunchy cereal (280 to 290)
½ cup steamed or boiled rice (85)	½ cup fried rice without meat (185)	½ cup rice pudding (235)
1 slice of bread (55 to 70)	1 corn muffin (125)	1 Danish pastry (275)
½ cup cooked noodles (100)	6 cheese ravioli with sauce (175)	1 cup lasagna (345)

Milk and Cheese Group

Lower	In-Between	Higher
½ cup (single dip) ice milk (95)	½ cup (single dip) ice cream (135)	1 cup vanilla milkshake (255)
1 oz. Cheddar cheese (115)	1 cup cheese souffle (260)	1 cup macaroni and cheese (430)
8 fl. oz. carton plain lowfat yogurt (145)	8 fl. oz. carton vanilla flavored yogurt (195)	8 fl. oz. carton yogurt with fruit or 2 dips frozen yogurt (225 to 240)

Meat, Poultry, Fish, and Beans Group

Lower	In-Between	Higher
2 oz. broiled chicken (95)	½ fried chicken breast (2¾ oz.) or 2 drumsticks (2½ oz.) (160 to 180)	8 oz. individual chicken pot pie (505)

3 oz. lean hamburger (without bun) (185)	3 oz. regular hamburger (without bun) (235)	3½ oz. cheeseburger (without bun) (320)
3 oz. lean roast beef (205)	3 oz. Swiss steak (315)	⅔ cup beef stroganoff over noodles (525)
2½ oz. broiled cod with butter or margarine (120)	2½ oz. fried, breaded ocean perch (160)	2½ oz. baked stuffed fish (½ cup bread stuffing) (325)
½ cup boiled navy beans (95)	1 cup navy bean soup (170)	1 cup baked navy beans (310)
3 oz. boiled shrimp (100)	3 oz. fried breaded shrimp (190)	½ cup shrimp Newburg (285)

The "Sweets" Group

Lower	In-Between	Higher
1 teaspoon sugar (15)	2 tablespoons pancake syrup (120)	12 fl. oz. cola (145)
3 oz. popsicle (70)	½ cup (single dip) sherbet (135)	1.2 oz. milk chocolate candy bar (175)

CALORIE COUNTDOWN MENUS

1200 calories	1800 calories	2400 calories

Breakfast

Orange juice, ½ cup	Orange juice, ¾ cup	Orange juice, 1 cup

Bran flakes with raisins, ½ cup	Bran flakes with raisins, ½ cup	Bran flakes with raisins, ½ cup
Milk, whole, ½ cup	Milk, whole, ½ cup	Milk, whole, ½ cup
Whole-wheat toast, 1 slice	Whole-wheat toast, 1 slice	Whole-wheat toast, 1 slice
Coffee/Tea	Jelly, 2 tsp	Jelly, 1 tbsp
	Coffee/Tea	Coffee/Tea

Lunch

Sandwich:	Sandwich:	Sandwich:
Ham, 2 ounces	Ham, 2 ounces	Ham, 2 ounces
Cheese, 1 slice (1 oz.)	Cheese, 1 slice (1 oz.)	Cheese, 1 slice (1 oz.)
Lettuce	Lettuce	Lettuce
Tomato, ½ medium	Tomato, ½ medium	Tomato, ½ medium
Enriched bread, 2 slices	Enriched bread, 2 slices	Enriched bread, 2 slices
Apple, 1 medium	Salad dressing, 2 tsp	Salad dressing, 2 tsp
Coffee/Tea	Apple, 1 medium	Apple, 1 medium
	Coffee/Tea	Plain cookies, 4
		Coffee/Tea

Dinner

Beef roast, 3 ounces	Beef roast, 4 ounces	Beef roast, 5 ounces
Baked potato, 1 medium	Baked potato, 1 medium	Baked potato, 1 medium
Broccoli, ½ cup	Broccoli, ½ cup	Broccoli, ½ cup
Milk, skim, 1 cup	Roll, 1	Roll, 1
	Margarine, 1 tsp	Margarine, 2 tsp
	Milk, lowfat (1%), 1 cup	Milk, lowfat (2%), 1 cup
	Angelfood cake (1/16), with strawberries, ½ cup	Angelfood cake (1/12), with strawberries, ½ cup and ice milk, ⅓ cup

Snacks

Cucumber slices,	Peach, fresh	Peach, fresh,

1 small cucumber   1 medium   1 medium
Carrot sticks,   Fruit-flavored yogurt,
  3-4 strips   1 cup
  (2½″ to 3″ long)   Banana, 1 small

SUGGESTED BODY WEIGHTS*

Range of Acceptable Weight

Height (feet-inches)	Men (Pounds)	Women (Pounds)
4'10″		92-119
4'11″		94-122
5'0″		96-125
5'1″		99-128
5'2″	112-141	102-131
5'3″	115-144	105-134
5'4″	118-148	108-138
5'5″	121-152	111-142
5'6″	124-156	114-146
5'7″	128-161	118-150
5'8″	132-166	122-154
5'9″	136-170	126-158
5'10″	140-174	130-163
5'11″	144-179	134-168
6'0″	148-184	138-173
6'1″	152-189	
6'2″	156-194	
6'3″	160-199	
6'4″	164-204	

NOTE: Height without shoes; weight without clothes.
SOURCE: HEW conference on obesity, 1973.

TO IMPROVE EATING HABITS

- Eat slowly
- Prepare smaller portions
- Avoid "seconds"

If you need to lose weight, do so gradually. Steady loss of 1 to 2 pounds a week — until you reach your goal — is relatively safe and more likely to be maintained. Long-term success depends upon acquiring new and better habits of eating and exercise. That is perhaps why "crash" diets usually fail in the long run.

Do not try to lose weight too rapidly. Avoid crash diets that are severely restricted in the variety of foods they allow. Diets containing fewer than 800 calories may be hazardous. Some people have developed kidney stones, disturbing psychological changes, and other complications while following such diets. A few people have died suddenly and without warning.

*NUTRITION AND YOUR HEALTH, USDA, Home and Garden Bulletin No. 232, p. 8.

TO LOSE WEIGHT

- Increase physical activity
- Eat less fat and fatty foods
- Eat less sugar and sweets

Gradual increase of everyday physical activities like walking or climbing stairs can be very helpful. The chart below gives the calories used per hour in different activities.

APPROXIMATE ENERGY EXPENDITURE BY A 150 POUND PERSON IN VARIOUS ACTIVITIES*

Activity	Calories per hour
Lying down or sleeping	80
Sitting	100
Driving an automobile	120
Standing	140
Domestic work	180
Walking, 2½ mph	210

Bicycling, 5½ mph	210
Gardening	220
Golf; lawn mowing, power mower	250
Bowling	270
Walking, 3¾ mph	300
Swimming, ¼ mph	300
Square dancing, volleyball; roller skating	350
Wood chopping or sawing	400
Tennis	420
Skiing, 10 mph	600
Squash and handball	600
Bicycling, 13 mph	660
Running, 10 mph	900

SOURCE: Based on material prepared by Robert E. Johnson, M.D., Ph.D., and colleagues, University of Illinois.

*NUTRITION AND YOUR HEALTH, USDA, House and Garden Bulletin No. 232, p. 9.

Chapter 36

Nutrition

Nutrition is the process by which living things, both plants and animals, take in, absorb, and use food for growth and survival.

NUTRITION: FOOD AT WORK FOR YOU, a publication of the United States Department of Agriculture (USDA), Washington, 1978, states: "Nutrition is the food you eat and how the body uses it." This bulletin lists, on pages 3 and 4, a daily food guide, which sorts foods into four groups on the basis of their similarity in nutrient content. Each group has a special contribution toward an adequate diet.

1. The Meat Group

   Foods included: beef, veal, lamb, pork, liver, heart, kidney; poultry and eggs; fish and shellfish; alternates: dry beans, dry peas, lentils, nuts, peanuts, peanut butter.

   Amounts recommended: Choose two or more servings everyday. Count as a serving the following: two or three ounces of lean meat, poultry, or fish, all without bone; one egg; one-half cup of cooked, dry beans, dry peas, or lentils; or two tablespoons of peanut butter to replace one-half serving of meat.

   Page one states that meat, poultry, fish, and eggs are valued for protein which is needed for growth and repair of body tissues — muscle, organs, blood, skin, and hair. These foods also contribute iron and B vitamins.

2. The Vegetable-Fruit Group

Foods included: all fruits and vegetables. This guide stresses those that are valuable as sources of vitamin C and vitamin A, which are listed below.

Sources of Vitamin C: good sources-grapefruit or grapefruit juice; orange or orange juice; cantaloupe; guava; mango; papaya; raw strawberries; broccoli; brussels sprouts; green pepper; sweet red pepper. Fair sources: honeydew melon; lemon; tangerine; tangerine juice; watermelon; asparagus; cabbage; collards; garden cress; kale; mustard greens; potatoes and sweet potatoes cooked in the jacket; spinach; tomatoes or tomato juice; turnip greens.

Sources of vitamin A: dark green and deep-yellow vegetables and a few fruits including apricots, broccoli, cantaloupe, carrots, chard, collards, cress, kale, mango, persimmon, pumpkin, spinach, sweet potatoes, turnip greens and other dark-green leaves, and winter squash.

Amounts recommended; Choose four or more servings every day including one serving of a good source of Vitamin C and two servings of a fair source. Choose one serving, at least every other day, of a good source of Vitamin A. The remaining one to three servings may be any vegetable or fruit, including those that are valuable for Vitamin C and for Vitamin A. Count as one serving one-half cup of vegetable or fruit, or a portion as ordinarily served, such as one medium apple, banana, orange, or potato, half a medium grapefruit or cantaloupe, or the juice of one lemon.

Pages one and two state that fruits and vegetables are valuable sources of vitamins and minerals. Vitamin C is needed for healthy gums and body tissues. Vitamin A is important for growth, normal vision, and a healthy condition of the skin and other body surfaces.

3. The Milk Group

Foods included: milk — fluid whole, evaporated, skim, dry, buttermilk; cheese — cottage, cream, Cheddar-type, natural or process; ice cream.

Amounts recommended: Some milk every day for everyone. Recommended amounts are given below in terms of 8-ounce cups of whole fluid milk:

Children under 9 — 2 to 3 cups
Children 9 to 12 — 3 or more cups
Teenagers — 4 or more cups
Adults — 2 or more cups

Part or all of the milk may be fluid skim milk, buttermilk, evaporated milk, or dry milk.

Cheese or ice cream may replace part of the milk. The amount is based on calcium content. Portions of cheese and ice cream and their milk equivalents in calcium are as follows:

1-inch cube of Cheddar-type cheese equals ½ cup milk
½ cup cottage cheese equals ⅓ cup milk
2 tablespoons cream cheese equals 1 tablespoon milk
½ cup ice cream or ice milk equals ⅓ cup milk

Page two states that foods in the milk group are relied on to meet most of the calcium needs of the day. Milk is the leading source of calcium, which is needed for bones and teeth. Milk also provides protein, riboflavin, Vitamin A, if whole or fortified, and many other nutrients.

4. The Bread and Cereal Group

Foods included: all breads and cereals that are whole grain, enriched, or restored. Check labels to be sure. Specifically, this group includes breads, cooked cereals, ready-to-eat cereals, cornmeal, crackers, flour, grits, macaroni and spaghetti, noodles, rice, rolled oats, quick breads and other baked goods if made with whole-grain or enriched flour.

Amounts recommended: Choose four servings or more daily. Or, if no cereals are chosen, have an extra serving of breads and baked goods. Count as one serving one slice of bread, one ounce of ready-to-eat cereal; ½ to ¾ cup cooked cereal, cornmeal, grits, macaroni, noodles, rice, or spaghetti.

Page two states that the bread-cereal group, with its whole-grain and enriched bread and other cereal products, furnishes protein, iron, several of the B-vitamins, and food energy.

Other foods: Everyone will use some foods not specified in the four food groups. Such foods include unenriched, refined breads, cereals, flours, sugars, butter, margarine, and other fats.[1]

Hundreds of bulletins are available from our government through agencies such as the United States Department of Agriculture and Health, Education and Welfare. All materials are in the public domain and may be used and shared freely. If you are interested in this remarkable service, a post card request will bring lists of materials available. Most are free. Some cost only a few pennies.

The address of the United States Department of Agriculture (USDA) is USDA, Washington, D.C. 20250. The Health, Education, and Welfare is HEW, 5600 Fishers Lane, Rockville, Maryland 20857.

Outstanding publications of the USDA include NUTRITION: FOOD AT WORK FOR YOU; DIETARY GUIDELINES OF AMERICANS, February, 1980; A PRIMER ON NUTRIENTS: Proteins, Carbohydrates, Fats, and Fiber (HEW); FOOD IS MORE THAN SOMETHING YOU EAT; FOOD: A PUBLICATION ON FOOD AND NUTRITION; and NUTRITION AND YOUR HEALTH: Dietary Guidelines for Americans.

Good nutrition cannot be overemphasized. In so many ways, it determines the way we look, the way we feel, and the way we think. It affects our lifespan!

For good physical and mental health, consider a balanced diet from the four food groups.

Chapter 37

Stress: A Dozen Ways to Combat It

S tress is a number-one health problem. High blood pressure, colitis, insomnia, gout, premenstrual tension, impotence, depression, ulcers, diabetes, headaches, allergies, infectious diseases, arthritis, and even cancer are often stress-related. Stress often leads to alcoholism, obesity, drug addiction, excessive smoking, divorce, accidents, and suicide.

Stress is with us to stay.

The all-important question is "What can we do about it?"

Efforts toward stress alleviation involve both physical and mental efforts.

Consider:

1. We do not breathe deeply enough, often enough. Sit straight. Breathe in through the nose, mouth closed. Hold for four counts. Then let air out slowly through the mouth. Do this several times. Feel refreshing strength and relief of fatigue.

2. Exercise stimulates the whole body and enhances deep breathing, improves blood circulation and heartbeat. Exercise is a natural tranquilizer. Try it. Run, jump rope,

climb stairs. Do calisthenics. Concerning depression, exercise works.

3. Eat right. Practice good nutrition. Eat something from the four food groups each day. Avoid certain foods that may cause stress — coffee, colas, teas, chocolate, and especially meats and other foods containing salt.

    The average daily diet should include about 85 grams of protein (best sources: poultry and fish), 350 grams of carbohydrates (fruits, vegetables, flour and cereal products), 55 grams of fat (fish and vegetable sources preferred), and 5 grams of fiber.

    Consider a daily vitamin tablet which is formulated to fight stress, one that contains minerals and iron. Minerals such as calcium, zinc, iodine, and sodium help to combat stress.

    The recommended dietary allowance for vitamin A (1000 milligrams per day), vitamin C (60 milligrams), and vitamin E (10 milligrams), is set by the Nutrition Board of the National Academy of Science National Research Council.

4. Think, plan, and discipline yourself to control time, as the chapter on "Time" advocates. Jot notes. Have a plan, no matter how simple. Keep a pad and pencil in strategic home areas where you work most, in the car, on your desk, in your handbag. Do not get a headache or get distressed trying to remember all you must do. Make hurried notes instead.

5. Make maximum use of your mind to think, to meditate. That may sound like a contradiction, but meditation does involve a concentrated effort in thinking relaxation. Simply sit down. Fold your hands in your lap. Put your feet up or under you, whatever is comfortable. Breathe deeply, but quietly. Think quietness, peace, stillness. Relax every part of your body from head to toe.

6. Do something really happy. Go for a walk on the mall, buy something personal or frivolous, not necessarily expensive, just for yourself. Try a new magazine, a book on self-improvement, a new lipstick. Consider a pot plant of

greenery or blossoms for your home — and you. Anything! Even a short car ride away from home, if only around the block, helps. It is amazing what momentary change can do for the psyche. Take a long, hot bath. Eat a good meal. Put clean sheets on the bed, sprinkle them with bath powder, and go to bed just after sundown. Turn down the sound on the phone and bribe a family member to answer all calls.

7. As the problem-solving chapter promises, "Even this shall pass away." Change is certain. A situation may be permanent, like the loss of a loved one or the loss of a limb, but environment and emotional influences will change. Tell yourself this again and again. A spokesman for the Food and Drug Administration stated that over ten million Americans take the artificial tranquilizer, valium. Search diligently for nature's way, for God's way.

8. Do something for someone.

9. Take a nap.

10. Talk to a friend.

11. Read.

12. Pray.

Part III

ETERNAL BEAUTY

The Ultimate Crowning

Chapter 38

Reaching Beyond Ourselves

Matthew 5:48 challenges us to "Be ye therefore perfect, even as your Father which is in heaven is perfect." Because we are physical beings in a physical world, not spiritual beings in a spiritual world, we interpret this Scripture as a challenge, not a command—for no one can obtain perfection in our world. Romans 3:10 emphasizes this with the words: "As it is written, There is none righteous, no, not one."

Yet, the challenge is always before us — to live the best we can, to learn all that we can, to do all that we can, to think all we can, to pray all we can — for others and for the glory of God. In so doing, almost without exception, we grow, we change, we mature in the Christian faith; and as Catherine Marshall wrote, we reach that realm where our souls, spirits, and beings reach a realm "beyond ourselves" — a place where we find a closer communion with God than we have ever known before. Robert Browning, the English poet, expressed the idea in this way when he wrote: "Ah, but a man's reach should exceed his grasp, or what's a heaven for?"

In America, in the middle 1800's, a group of brilliant young men led by Ralph Waldo Emerson, emphasized the idea of transcendentalism — a philosophy that mind goes beyond matter and that man can know more than he really sees or experiences. In other words, Emerson and others believed that through thought, prayer, study, and concentrated effort, man can go beyond himself to come in contact with Divine truth. Many transcendentalists thought that true spirit had gone out of the churches and that religion needed new inspiration and new vision.

Even though we, as Christians, may not accept all the teachings of the transcendentalists, their ideas of man's continuous, in-depth search for truth, for right, for good, and for God, are worthy of our sincerest consideration.

Perhaps there is not one of us who has not looked at the life of another and wondered: "What makes him, or her, 'tick'?" The answer to this is that it may be talent, or training, a gift from God, or a special blessing. Yet, on the other hand, that special insight or ability, or "know-how" may be the result of constant striving to seek, to find, to learn. It may come from that special effort to find, to memorize, to recall a great idea, or to read about great people in the Bible and in the world to see what made them "tick."

You will recall that not too many months ago, on the reverse side of highway ice-warning signs, was written the word "think." On one occasion, my dad remarked that he thought that the word *think* was one of the most powerful words in our language.

Yet, how often do we really think? How often do we recall the thoughts of the Bible, the ideas of a sermon, the meaning of a great quotation, the depth of spoken idea to make it a part of our conscious or subconscious mind? It is often so much easier to let things come and go and pass away without making them a part of us daily — or when we need them for inspiration, sharing, or transcending!

In most of our local schools each year at graduation, two seniors are given a small, but powerful, book given by the Danforth Foundation entitled "I Dare You." This little volume challenges its readers to fourfold development: Think Tall, Stand Tall, Smile Tall, and Live Tall. The book emphasizes that we have not one life to live, but four: a body (Physical), a brain (Mental), a heart (Social), and a soul (Spiritual).

In St. Paul's Cathedral, London, on a tablet to the memory of General Charles Gordon, we find these immortal words:

> "He at all times and everywhere gave
> His Strength to the Weak
> His Substance to the Poor
> His Sympathy to the Suffering
> His Heart to God."

In reality, these words express truthfully what life is all about. Yet, somewhere, somehow, if we can learn, through praying, studying, Bible reading, loving others and God, and thinking deeply about good, inspiring, beautiful things, maybe we can come in even greater contact with Divine truth and power to be even more what God would have us to be.[1]

Chapter 39

It Takes Only One

The number "one" is the smallest unit of numerical measure. Yet, it may, in many respects, be considered the largest, for it often represents the highest, the greatest, the best! This little number is truly a paradox if we have one penny, generally we feel that we do not have much; if our team is "number one," we feel that it is tops.

One makes a difference. Consider these:

1. It takes only one word, spoken to a young person, to change his destiny.
2. One step, one gesture, or one word, "forgive," to rebuild a marriage.
3. One quiet word to calm a mob.
4. One move in the right direction, at the right moment, to save a life.

On the other hand, consider these:

1. It takes only one hastily-spoken, careless, profane word to tarnish a personality.
2. One inconsiderate, bitter person to create enough confusion, frustration, and misunderstanding to split a church.

3. One thoughtless act to ruin a character.
4. One angry bullet to snatch away a life.
5. One careless driver to maim innocent bodies for life.
6. One button pushed by a maniac to destroy a civilization.

In 1692, nineteen people lost their lives by being burned at the stake in the Salem witchcraft trials because of the foolishness of one young girl, Ann Putnam, who accused women of being witches. She stirred people, through a West Indian named Tituba, to believe that the accused women were actually witches.

According to a recent sermon by the Rev. Billy Graham, one mechanical defect caused 346 people to lose their lives in a plane crash in France.

Recently, in a hospital in our state, a young woman with serious facial injuries lay on a narrow operating table where she was given a piece of gauze to wipe the blood as she watched the other injured persons as they were brought into the emergency room — broken, bleeding, and screaming. It takes only one person.

Animals awaiting slaughter at slaughter houses suffer from hunger, thirst, and crowding. It takes only one person to change such as this!

On March 25, 1976, the front page headline of the WILSON DAILY TIMES was "1975 Crime Rate Rose 9 Percent." This change in the crime rate began with one person.

Consider for a moment, the blessings of such people as Abraham, Moses, Joseph, and Paul; of people like the Revs. Billy Graham, Billy Sunday, and Albert Schweitzer; of doctors, nurses, and teachers; of friends; of mothers, daddies, and countless others. One person makes a difference!

Most important of all:

1. It took only one God to give His only begotten Son.
2. One Christ Jesus to die to save a world of millions.
3. One idea, "love," put into action, to change a world.
4. One act, "faithfulness," to reap a destiny.
5. One word, "well-done," to find an eternity.

Chapter 40

It Takes Only Five Minutes

A few days ago a friend told me about a relative who had praised her because she was able to keep her knife-fork-and-spoon drawer in order. The friend related that she had consoled the relative by saying, "Well, we can't do everything," but then added, "but you know, it takes fewer than five minutes a day to keep a silverware drawer in order."

There is great truth in that statement, and even greater reality lies in the truth that it takes only five minutes to do many things.

> It takes only five minutes to call an aged, ill, or depressed friend, or to make a just-to-keep-in-touch-because-I-care call.
>
> It takes only five minutes to write a cheerful note, and even less time to write a card or to sign a greeting card.
>
> It takes only five minutes to talk with a child about a problem — or a dream.
>
> It takes only five minutes to say, "How are you today?" "Are you troubled?" or "Is something bothering you?" — and to listen to an answer.

It takes only five minutes to read a chapter in the Bible, and less time to read a few verses.

It takes only five minutes to add fresh flowers to a room, or to write a note of praise to leave on a child's pillow.

Moreover,

It takes only five seconds to be born into life: it takes fewer than five seconds to be borne unto eternity.

It takes only one second to say, "I love you," to a yearning, hungry heart.

It takes only one second to say, "Forgive me."

It takes only one second to say, "Help me."

It takes only one second to say, "I love you, God."

Most of all, it takes only a split second to say a one-word prayer by breathing that holy name, JESUS.

A split second is all we really need.

A split second will someday be all we have.

Chapter 41

Sometimes We Stand Alone

Man is by nature gregarious. God created him with a natural desire to be with others. Even though the creation of man and woman is recorded in Genesis 1:26, God emphasizes a strong, universal motive when Genesis 2:18 states: "And the Lord said, It is not good that man should be alone; I will make him an help meet for him." The key word is *alone*. God did not want man to be alone. ". . . It is not good . . ." He said.

Yet, loneliness is one of the key problems in America today. In all walks of life, there is the pounding of the heartbeat to the rhythm of David's words: ". . . No man cared for my soul" (Psalm 142:4). Teenagers are afraid of the future. Divorce figures, job losses, and unexpected illnesses tear into the lives of the young as well as the middle-aged who have already faced family problems of alcohol, drugs, and sacrifical survival. The old sit in rest homes, hospitals, or at home — alone somewhere with only the strength to stare and stumble. People with cancer, heart problems, mental illness, and other similar concerns lie lonely in hospital beds only to wonder and wait.

Life challenges us to be positive. The Bible teaches us to look up and live. Yet, life is the stark reality of human existence — looking at life as it really is! This brings us to know that at times we must stand alone: we must make decisions and face realities which are overwhelming and overpowering.

Research would prove to us that almost all of the Biblical people stood alone at one time or another: Moses on the Mount, Joseph before Pharaoh, Paul before Agrippa, Stephen before his stoners, Jesus before Pilate.

How often we are called upon to stand alone! No one can help us or tell us what to do. We face a financial crisis, a serious illness, a fatal disease, the plague of being misunderstood or misquoted, the weariness of chronic fatigue, the sight of a closed casket, and we cry the words of the Cross: "My God, why hast thou forsaken me?" (Matthew 27:46). We weep in the night and say, "Please, God, help me. I've gone the last mile of the way!" We ask over and over the eternal question of Job: "Why, God? Why?"

There is no answer. The why of human suffering and aloneness is an unanswerable question that transcends the ability of man to comprehend. Some things belong to God. Our greatest challenge is to live so close to God that we feel that whatever happens is within His divine will. And constantly, with Him, we make decisions, and then live with the hope: "I did the best I knew to do."

Perhaps we can find comfort in these words by Eugenia Price: "It could be that the shared silence is His way of teaching us the language of Eternity."

Further, as we reach to others who are lonely, she poses this thought-provoking question: "Have we eaten so much cake and drunk so much coffee in the church fellowship halls that we have forgotten the Man of Galilee who was often hungry and had no place to lay His head?"

The answer to loneliness may be found in hearing the lonely cry of another. It has something to do with tuning our ears to hear the guidance of "that still small Voice."

Constantly, in our human frailty, we must remind ourselves that "He walks with me and He talks with me, and He tells me I am His own. And the joy we share as we tarry there, none other has ever known."

So, like the aging trees of the wayside, we often stand alone — battered, broken, bent. We stand alone, except for God!

Chapter 42

O Lord, God, Help Us to Find Our Way

W e are idealists: we are dreamers! And we should be! We want the newest, the best, the loveliest. But life is not always that way. It often calls us to realism.

Tragedy, trouble, and trauma are all about us. How often have we seen destruction, or felt similar ravagement in our own lives.

A well-known weekly recently featured a multi-page centerfold on stress. The U.S. NEWS, March 21, 1977, featured the same subject. One writer described stress as the number one health problem.

When trouble comes, we, in our human forms, must face it and try to overcome it. To the followers of the Master of Galilee, the ways are obvious: faith, hope, prayer, Bible study, and love. We must walk hand in hand with God to help solve our problems.

Yet, there is an adage which says: ''Heaven helps those who help themselves.''

One way to help ourselves is through our thoughts. Paraphrasing John Milton, we are reminded that ''The mind within itself can make a heaven of torment or a torment of heaven." Consider: If sometimes we don't get lost, we may never find our way. An Old German Proverb says: "Take life as it happens, but try to make it happen the way you want to take it." We cannot control what happens to us oftentimes, but we can often control the way we react and overcome.

Another way that we can help ourselves is by trying never to look back, at least, not to look back with regrets. Robert Frost expressed this idea in a poem in which he faced the choice of two roads. He wrote: "Two roads diverged into a wood and I — I took the one less traveled by, and that has made all the difference. . . ." Paul said so beautifully in Philippians 3:13, 14 — ". . . Forgetting those things which are behind . . . I press toward the mark for the prize of the high calling of God in Christ Jesus." There are times when we must pick up the broken pieces, and leave, except for an occasional memory, that which is lost and build on that which is left.

In times of trouble or happiness, we should consider following the unfollowed path, blazing a trail to someone or something good or right. Muriel Strade wrote: "I will not follow where the path may lead, but I will go where there is no path, and I will leave a trail." Remember, as Charles Spurgeon said: "Faith goes up the stairs that love has made and looks out the windows which hope has opened," and "Love weighs more than gold" (Josephine Bacon).

Even as our lives are shattered and torn, we must try constantly to remember, as the Oriental Proverb teaches: "Rejoice at life, for the time is more advanced than we think." Helen Keller, our blind inspiration wrote: "Keep your face to the sunshine and you cannot see the shadow." Erasmus penned: "Give light and the darkness will disappear."

Most of all, at all times, we must keep our eyes turned to that Eternal Light, remembering, as an unknown writer expressed: "When He came, there was no light: when He left, there was no darkness."

Chapter 43

Turning Aside to the Quiet Roads

A few days ago, in the late afternoon, I traveled from Wilson to the heart of Durham almost without stopping my car, not even for a stoplight. After one leaves Wilson, the remaining miles are a steady effort of hurry-up-and-go, passing, watching for on-coming travelers, or keeping out of the way of faster-moving vehicles.

Business in Durham was quickly finished and the return trip began. It was a rainy, hazy Friday afternoon. Weary workers scurried home, and drivers of big trucks seemed to be putting forth special effort for that last minute push toward an important destination.

Finally, I reached Wilson again. Leaving highway 264, I drove down 301 to the place where I was to turn again to travel quieter, calmer roads.

This is not an unusual experience, for all of us, and hundreds of others make similar trips daily or often.

Yet, as I turned off 301, I was reminded of the spiritual truth that we need to leave the hurrying, scurrying world of action and activity to review and renew our lives in the quiet places on quieter roads.

How good it was to leave the noise of the big trucks, the swishing of passing cars, the smell of fuel fumes, and the fear of possible accidents. I could actually feel the tension leave my body.

How often in our busy, hurried, noisy, fearful lives do we need to turn aside to the "be calm roads." A favorite verse of Scripture is "Be still, and know that I am God: . . ." (Psalm 46:10). How good it is to turn again to the calm, pleasant paths through meditation, rest, communion, stillness, and again, quietness.

There is beauty and inspiration in the quiet life. Serenity, stillness, and silence are attributes worth striving for. Many verses of Scripture challenge us to this philosophy. "He maketh the storm a calm, so that the waves thereof are still. Then are they glad because they are quiet; . . ." (Psalm 107:29, 30). "The whole earth is at rest, and is quiet: . . ." (Isaiah 14:7). Most of all, verses from our beloved Twenty-Third Psalm inspire us: "He maketh me to lie down in green pastures: he leadeth me beside the still waters. He restoreth my soul: . . ."

Noise pollution is a vital problem in America. The Federal Government is so concerned that it recently passed a law saying that the maximum noise level that a person can be exposed to for an eight-hour period cannot exceed 80 decibels. The street corners of New York constantly register 70 decibels; a jack hammer 150, and big trucks, 80-90.

Constant, rapid motion, as well as noise, surrounds us. Even in many human situations, especially in groups, there seems to be overwhelming loudness and restlessness. Uncontrolled voices and actions that create noise seem to be the popular practice. Even in homes, loud-playing televisions, radios, hi-fi's, and stereos crash constantly and loudly through the air.

In the March, 1976, issue of GOOD HOUSEKEEP-ING, Dr. Herbert Benson recommends six steps toward relaxation. Transcendental meditation, yoga, and relaxation therapy, as well as tranquilizers and suppressants, are the mode of the day.

Yet, there is a deeper, stronger, more certain quietness that reaches to the depth of human needs to bring an eternal peace that reaches to the very core of the human heart as well as the human spirit. Again, it is found in these words: "Be still, and know that I am God," and in the beautiful invitation, "Come unto me, all ye that labour and are heavy laden, and I will give you rest. Take my yoke upon you, and learn of me; for I am meek and lowly in heart: and ye shall find rest unto your souls" (Matthew 11:28, 29). To do this is to capture the secret of calmness and quietness, for now and for the eternal.

Chapter 44

Finding My Place Amid the Throng

I shared with you my thoughts concerning noise pollution and jet speed in the chapter, "Turning Aside to the Quiet Roads." We considered the thought, "Be still, and know that I am God: . . ." (Psalm 46:10).

There are, among our population, many who are caught in the noisy confusion of life, and who choose, eventually, if only temporarily, to seek the quiet ways.

On the other hand, though, this thought bears an interesting paradox: One needs "to get away from it all." Yet, many are so destined that they need "to get involved in it all" — even if for a little while.

How many of us have become so weary and lonely and discouraged that we simply get into our cars to drive around the block or to ride uptown for just a few minutes?

Moreover, how many of us have visited a hospital, a rest home, or a mental institution, only to return home to count our blessings more than ever? How many have stood on a busy street corner, or watched the masses from a tall building window, or a parked car, only to bow our head in prayerful concern for human life? Illness, age, rebellion, poverty, abuse, and neglect afflict our human race.

We return to our quiet place, alone, thankful. Thankful, yes, for many things. But not happy! For gradually, if not suddenly, there comes a restlessness. We recall the great truths: "For every man shall bear his own burden" (Galatians 6:5). This reminds us that each man, in his own way, must find God. Further, though, we realize, "Bear ye one another's burdens, . . ." (Galatians 6:2); the Great Commission, ". . . Go ye into all the world, . . ." (Mark 16:15); and the great challenge, ". . . Go out into the highways and hedges, . . ." (Luke 14:23).

Then we see the great paradox, the extremes which are opposite, yet both are great truths: We need, and seek, the quiet ways; yet, we need, and seek, to be our brother's keeper.

"How?" we ask.

The answer is obvious. It involves desire and determination, prayer and purpose, love and loyalty, searching and sacrifice, care and concern.

Perhaps the answer lies in four words which capture the meaning of our needs: first, "Be still, . . ."; then "Go ye. . . ."

Chapter 45

Tarnished Trophies

"Nothing is ever as good as it seems beforehand. Nothing!" These are the words of Nancy to Godfrey in George Eliot's great novel entitled SILAS MARNER.

How true these words are. Have you ever planned a vacation or trip, only to be disappointed once you reach your destination? Have you ever sacrificed for a new dress or suit or car, only to feel let down a few hours after the purchase?

The Bible calls us to service and to stewardship — to give of our best to the Master. Herein lies one of the greatest challenges to Christians. In our work for Him, we must be careful not to become engrossed in motives and attitudes so that we become obsessed by goals and gain, rewards and recognition. This leads to selfishness, covetousness and greed. History records, and newspapers report daily, the supreme sacrifices of character, reputation, and good will that are exchanged for a moment of glory or success. Benjamin Franklin wrote: "He has paid dear, very dear, for tne whistle." How true this is when we let blind ambition drive us regardless of whom we hurt or the price we pay.

Success, fame, recognition, glory, and praise must not be sought as a goal or an end. Success must be a natural, normal outgrowth of God's goodness and grace as we work hand in hand with Him to do His will.

I am constantly inspired by Rudyard Kipling's thought: "God gives all men all earth to love." There are enough opportunities and spaces for service in God's great, wide, wonderful world so that we need not tread on the life of another to achieve or serve.

Families have been torn asunder, churches have been split, and the happiness of countless lives has been destroyed because someone was driven by an obsession for leadership, recognition, or praise — or maybe a job or position that God had already given to another.

I am constantly reminded of the New York hero who turned to a friend and said: "Today it's me; tomorrow it will be somebody else." Think of how fleeting and fragile are fame and glory.

Trophies are beautiful and they glitter in the sunlight. But they tarnish! Martin Luther penned these beautiful words: "I have held many things in my hands, and I have lost them all; but whatever I have placed in God's hands, that I still possess."

Perhaps we could supplement George Eliot's words and say: "Nothing is ever so good as it seems beforehand. Nothing, except heaven!" And if we travel with clean hands and pure hearts, even the journey is beautiful!

Chapter 46

What, Then, Is an Education?

T housands of young people graduate from the high
school and colleges of our land. It is a time of joy
and of achievement.

Solomon valued wisdom above all things. "Wisdom
is the principal thing; therefore get wisdom: and with all
thy getting, get understanding" (Proverbs 4:7). Yet, it
was not a formal education or knowledge or facts that
Solomon sought, but understanding through a percep-
tive mind that enabled him to think wisely and deeply. It
is true that reading, thinking, listening, and learning
help to discipline and to train the human mind for
thought and depth of understanding; but learning without common sense and love almost always produces an
unbecoming personality and character.

The Bible warns against pride, snobbery, and conceit
— the "educated fool," as we often hear it expressed:
". . . it is written, I will destroy the wisdom of the wise,
and will bring to nothing the understanding of the pru-
dent. Where is the wise? . . . hath not God made foolish
the wisdom of the world?" (1 Corinthians 1:19, 20).

Also, "Let no man deceive himself. If any man among you seemeth to be wise in this world, let him become a fool, that he may be wise. For the wisdom of the world is foolishness with God. . . . And again, The Lord knoweth the thoughts of the wise, that they are vain" (1 Corinthians 3:18-20).

Over 200 verses of Scripture refer to the word "wisdom." Will you agree with me that Solomon would have said that wisdom is knowing the will of God and doing it? "Get wisdom, get understanding: forget it not; neither decline from the words of my mouth. Forsake her not, and she shall preserve thee: love her, and she shall keep thee" (Proverbs 4:5, 6).

In education, consider the value of an open mind, consideration of new ideas, getting along with people, constant learning, listening to others, willingness to work, worthy ambition, appreciation for the good and beautiful, and perpetuation of truth and faith.

Louisa Mae Alcott wrote: "There is virtue in country houses, fields, gardens, orchards, streams, and groves; in rustic recreation and plain manners that neither cities nor universities enjoy."

Maybe the answer lies in the thought that it takes it all — Bible, books, school, knowledge, living, and loving — all that we can learn and find and do and be to truly love God and others sincerely and purely.

Again, we turn to our Perfect Example: ". . . Jesus increased in wisdom and stature, and in favour with God and man" (Luke 2:52).

The challenge is always with us: "So teach us to number our days, that we may apply our hearts unto wisdom" (Psalm 90:12).

Chapter 47

If You Love Me, Please Tell My Mother

Recently, I was telling one of my library assistants how grateful I was for all she had done, and what a blessing she had been to my life through her work, attitude, and devotion. She looked at me seriously, and when I had finished, with tears in her eyes, she said, "If you love me, please tell my mother."

I did tell her mother. I wrote, among other things, "If I had a daughter like Cathy, how proud and grateful I would be. To have a daughter like Cathy is not to have lived in vain."

Perhaps we can think of at least one mother that we could make happy by writing her a message about a worthy daughter.

We need to be concerned about the mothers of others — all mothers — for they have made our churches, our homes, and our land good and great. But then, there comes that all-important question: "What shall I do for my own dear mother this year?"

What about considering these:

1. Promise to call her once a week. Or don't promise her,

just start doing it every Thursday night, and soon she'll expect it and look forward to it. For many of us, this will cost only 25 cents per week. That is just a fraction over one dollar per month, or thirteen dollars a year. Where can you buy such a gift for such a price?

2. Go to see her once a week, or once a day, if possible — not just for Sunday dinner! For many, this takes only a few minutes and means so much.

3. Write her a letter every week. It can contain news, words of gratitude, and love. Do you know the joy of going to the mailbox to find a personal letter from someone you love? Moreover, do you know the emptiness of finding only a newspaper and a bunch of impersonal circulars? A letter a week costs only $9.36 per year. Where can you buy a gift like that for that price?

4. Take her a flower and plant it in her yard. Too, sneak over to her house one day and mow the yard, trim the shrubs, or chop the borders.

5. Make a little corsage and give it to her on her birthday — or any day. She has given us so many "roses"; how many have we given her?

6. Write a little poem of love or a short letter. Frame it and give it to her. She'll cherish it.

7. Find a tiny souvenir, such as a small article of clothing or a wee toy from among her grandchildren's things, and give these to her. (I'd rather have a gift of love that someone has used or handled or worn or shared than to have a "store-bought" one any day.)

8. Fix her a little box (or a big box) of personal things that she would not buy for herself — hand lotion, bath powder, nail clippers — a "great big bunch" of surprises.

9. Buy her groceries for her one week. Leave them on the back porch like Santa Claus. Include some things she wouldn't dare buy for herself.

10. Take time to go places together — not just to get groceries, to the doctor, or shopping. Go for a ride just to talk or visit a friend or to get an ice-cream cone. "Waste" a little time together. It will be your most valuable memory in days to come!

If your mother is no longer living, find a mother whose children are far away and visit her. Visit an aged mother or one who is in a rest home or who lives alone. Talk to her, listen to her, hold her close before you leave. Hundreds of older people are starving for the feeling of a loving touch from someone who cares. Just look. You'll find one who needs you.

So often we think of tangible, concrete gifts, and they are important. Could we not, however, consider this year the gift of a prayer — a prayer for our mother everyday? Could we not make this, too, a prayer for forgiveness — forgiveness for our indifference, our ingratitude, and our neglect — with a prayer that God will give us strength and courage to be more devoted?

Could we not, too, include Daddy in all this? "Mom" and "Dad" are one, you know. God made them so when He joined them together in holy matrimony.

In His dying moments, Jesus looked at John and said, as He spoke of His own mother who stood at the foot of the Cross: ". . . Woman, behold thy son! . . . Behold thy mother! . . ." (John 19:26, 27).

Can we not perpetuate this great request as we "behold our own dear mother"?

Chapter 48

Daddy Does the Lights

When I complimented a group of students from our school on their production of "Yankee Doodle," a young man, with eyes sparkling, said, "You didn't see me, but I helped, too. I was behind the curtains. I did the lights."

How much this is like fathers, I thought. They often stay behind the scenes and do the lights!

There is something sacred about the word "father." William Wordsworth said: "Father! — to God himself we cannot give a holier name."

When I think of an ideal mother, I recall verses from Proverbs 31. When I think of an appropriate tribute to an ideal father, I turn first of all to Psalm 1: "Blessed is the man that walketh not in the counsel of the ungodly, nor standeth in the way of sinners, nor sitteth in the seat of the scornful. But his delight is in the law of the LORD; and in his law doth he meditate day and night. And he shall be like a tree planted by the rivers of water, that bringeth forth his fruit in his season; his leaf also shall not wither; and whatsoever he doeth shall prosper" (Psalm 1:1-3).

A few years ago, the National Father's Day Committee suggested these guideposts for fathers: "A wise father encourages respect for other nations, gives a child confidence through a happy home, teaches a child that he is no better than others, and is quick to offer a helping hand in time of trouble." Further, the committee suggested that a good father "school his child in good sportsmanship and fair play, gain respect and love of his child not by force but through companionship and wisdom, teach his child the value of good citizenship and instill in him a respect for law and order, teach him that intolerance and ignorance are alien to a world of peace, and above all, through spiritual guidance, emphasize that greatness and goodness go hand in hand."

Because so many of us have fathers who work with the soil, the following poem by Katherine Edelman seems appropriate:

> My father has love of land:
> He often would reach his lean, brown hand,
> Curving his fingers to form a cup
> And draw a handful of rich soil up.
>
> I still can hear him, pride in his tone,
> "Be rightfully proud of the land you own."
>
> Then, with brown earth from his fingers spilled,
> Downward to furrows carefully tilled,
> He would say, his own wide fields in view:
> "Keep the land, and the land will keep you."

George Eliot wrote: "There are debts we can't pay like we pay money debts." Such are the debts we owe to our dad. We can pay and repay only in part. Perhaps the only thing we can truly do is to reach forth to others and upward to God to perpetuate those good and worthy things which our dad taught by word and example.

Robert Louis Stevenson wrote: "That man is a success who has lived well, laughed often, and loved much, who has gained the respect of intelligent men and the love of children, who leaves the world better than he found it, and looked for the best in others as he gave the best he had." Most of all, that dad has not lived in vain who has, through a child's life, stood in the background or behind the scenes and "done the lights."

>Thank you, Daddy,
>>for food, raiment,
>>>and shelter,
>>for pennies, nickles,
>>>dimes, and dollars,
>>for fishing trips, for
>>>toys, for quiet walks
>>>and talks,
>>for medicine, sleepless
>>>nights, and your hand
>>>upon my forehead
>>>when I was ill.
>
>Thank you, Daddy,
>>for life, for love,
>>for labor;
>>for pain, for sacrifice,
>>for prayers,
>>for living a good, godly
>>>life — and teaching me
>>>to do the same.
>
>Thank you, Daddy,
>>for all you have done
>>>and been,
>>>>and patiently,
>>>>willingly,
>>>>>unfalteringly
>>>>>>given —
>>All for me!

—Joyce Proctor Beaman

Chapter 49

Regrets

I have often heard my dad say that one of the main
regrets of his life was that he did not have enough
time to spend with us children when we were young.
During those Depression days and war years, when
labor was very scarce, with farm work, custom work for
the neighbors, caring for the livestock morning and
night, and other duties, he often left us in bed when he
went to work in the fields and did not return until we
were asleep again in the evening. I always assured him
that it was not the quantity of time spent with us, but the
quality — and the quality was always good. But he
never seemed quite satisfied.

If someone were to ask, "What is the chief regret of
your life?" what would your answer be? Because we
are physical beings, not spiritual ones, I am sure that the
answers would be numerous for each individual and
that all of us would have regrets.

We may regret that we do not read the Bible enough,
that we do not pray enough, or attend church so much
as we should. We regret that we do not take time to eat

properly and well, to think right, and to exercise regularly.

But I imagine that one of the main regrets would be that we do not spend enough time with friends, with other human lives that we love.

Jesus said, "This is my commandment, That ye love one another, as I have loved you." It is true that we can love in spirit, apart from one another, but fellowship in person is so much sweeter.

Friendship, like so many other good things, is an almost selfish experience because we receive so much more, oftentimes, than we are able to give. Robert Louis Stevenson said, "A friend is a present you give to yourself." But remember, if you crush rose petals in your palm, the fragrance will linger on the hand you clasp. So friendship is a two-way joy.

Emerson wrote: "A friend is a person with whom I can be sincere." What greater joy than another human life with whom I can be truthful, sincere, open, and uninhibited. An unknown author wrote: "There are two things that go into the make-up of friendship, the one is truth, the other is understanding."

Proverbs 18:24 states: "A man that hath friends must show himself friendly: and there is a friend that sticketh closer than a brother." Proverbs 17:17 says: "A friend loveth at all times," and John 15:13 challenges in all its beauty: "Greater love hath no man than this, that a man lay down his life for his friends."

Perhaps, with many other things, we need to stop to consider how the rush of our busy life has caused us to neglect our friends. We may be so busy that we cannot even at this moment visit a friend, but we can breathe this prayer which God's Spirit can take across the airways: "The Lord watch between me and thee, when we are absent one from another." (See Genesis 31:49.)

Or the Irish blessing: "May the road rise up to meet you, may the wind be ever at your back, may the sun shine warm upon your face, and rains fall soft upon your fields, and until we meet again, may God hold you in the palm of His hand."

Man is the ultimate of God's creation. Human life is sacred. A part of it, which we call the soul, is the only thing which time passes on to eternity. Therefore, when we link our life to that of another in spiritual friendship, this is honorable in the sight of God.

Especially, when we tune our lives to that Great Friend of Galilee, we touch the very heart of God.

Chapter 50

Dear God, Please Give Me One More Sunrise . . .

I have always been fascinated by the similarity of a sunrise and a sunset. Generally, by looking at a photo, one can hardly tell the difference.

For us, the sunrise is the beginning of the day. Yet, our sunset is the beginning of a new day for people in another part of the world. So a sunset is really part of an eternal, unbroken cycle or circle of sunrises.

So it is with life. There is really no sunset, for Jesus said, "I am Alpha and Omega, the beginning and the ending" (Revelation 1:8).

Somewhere between the sunrise and the sunset, for a brief span that we call years, there is light. And in that light we learn to live, to labor, and to laugh — to cry, to care, to cure. Most of all, somewhere between the sunrise and the sunset, before the darkness, we find love — for though we speak with the tongues of men and angels and have not love, we are as sounding brass or a tinkling cymbal (1 Corinthians 13:1).

As has so often been said, every day is a new chance,

a new opportunity — to begin again. Even every moment or every hour is thus! God, in His Divine plan, has given man many reminders of the blessing of starting again, of changing, of growing.

Charles DuBois wrote: "The important thing is this: to be able at any moment to sacrifice what we are for what we could become."

So often we say, "If only I had one more chance." In many things, we do not have a second chance; yet, in many things we do have another opportunity, if we would only take advantage of it. This may involve a denial of self or a casting away of false pride or burdening habits. Nevertheless, the chance is still there.

Are we not too often prone to let small, really insignificant things destroy our ability to function as a Christian and as a brother to man? Let us consider for a moment the time when that moment shall come, and we shall have one last chance to consider what is really important — when all that is left is that last prayer: "Dear God, give me one more sunrise," or even: "Let me spend my last sunset with You in that Great Eternal Sunrise."

Chapter 51

Faith

"Now faith is the substance of things hoped for,
the evidence of things not seen" (Hebrews 11:1).
THE HOLY BIBLE, King James Version

L ike hope and love, faith is another paradox: it is
both seen and unseen.

Of all the expressions of faith from the pen of man,
the following is perhaps the most all-inclusive except
for the Bible. This parable has been circulated widely in
recent years and has appeared in religious journals and
in newspaper columns such as Ann Landers. The author is unknown.

One Night I Had a Dream . . .

I dreamed I was walking along the beach with the Lord, and
across the sky flashed scenes from my life. For each scene I
noticed two sets of footprints in the sand; one belonged to me,
the other to the Lord. When the last scene of my life flashed
before us, I looked back at the footprints in the sand. I noticed
that many times along the path of my life, there was only one
set of footprints. I also noticed that it happened at the very

lowest and saddest times in my life. I questioned the Lord about it. "Lord, You said that once I decided to follow You, You would walk with me all the way. But I have noticed that during the most troublesome times in my life, there is only one set of footprints. I don't understand why in times when I needed You most, You would leave." The Lord replied, "My precious child, I would never leave you during your times of trial and suffering. When you see only one set of footprints, it was then that I carried you."

Chapter 52

One Solitary Life

Beyond the Bible, there is no literature more beautiful than the thoughts of "One Solitary Life," from the pen of an unknown writer. The truth of its message transcends all.

Always, when I have been asked to share thoughts with any organization, whenever possible, I have chosen to end with this masterpiece of beauty and truth. The pages of YOU ARE BEAUTIFUL: YOU REALLY ARE would be incomplete without it.

He was born in an obscure village,
the child of a peasant woman.
He grew up in still another village, where he worked
in a carpenter shop until he was thirty.
Then for three years he was an itinerant preacher.
He never wrote a book. He never held an office.
He never had a family or owned a house. He didn't
go to college. He never visited a big city.
He never traveled two hundred miles from the place
where he was born. He did none of the things
one usually associates with greatness.
He had no credentials but himself. He was only

thirty-three when the tide of public opinion
turned against him. His friends ran away. He was
turned over to his enemies and went through
the mockery of a trial. He was nailed to a cross
between two thieves. While he was dying,
his executioners gambled for his clothing,
the only property he had on earth.
When he was dead, he was laid in a borrowed grave
through the pity of a friend.
Nineteen centuries have come and gone, and today
he is the central figure of the human race
and the leader of mankind's progress.
All the armies that ever marched, all the navies
that ever sailed, all the parliaments that ever sat,
all the kings that ever reigned, put together,
have not affected the life of man
on this earth as much at that
ONE SOLITARY LIFE.
Author Unknown

Chapter 53

Does She Think That She Is Beautiful?

In an earlier book, I wrote that compassion is a most-
desired attribute, for like love, it encompasses all.
Hand in hand with compassion is honesty.

Consider the man whose word is his bond and his
promise his sacred honor: a man who pays his debts and
figures his "just wages."

Obsession with honesty is admirable and desirable.

Many times, as you have read this book, you may
have asked, "Does she think she is beautiful?"

Such a question must remain rhetorical.

We leave that labeling to you, to others, and to God.

Daily, we say to ourselves:

> This is a task that I must do.
> This is a quality that I must improve.
> This is a trait that I must polish.
> This is a habit that I must change.

Constantly, quietly, day-by-day, we go about our
work in our homes and in our professions, silently
seeking to the preservation and perpetuation of those
gifts and blessings that God has given to us. Unaware,

we become: unaware, we are! It is as spontaneous as a smile, as unrehearsed as a prayer. The praise belongs to God — and to those who love us.

I suppose if I could choose my epitaph, I would cast my lot with James Henry Leigh Hunt when he wrote in "Abou Ben Adhem": ". . . Write me as one that loves his fellow-men."

That is why I wrote this book.

I wrote it for you — because I love you.

And you are beautiful . . . You really are!

Chapter 54

You Are Beautiful When You Walk with God

"And I said to the man who stood at the gate of the year:
  'Give me a light that I may tread safely into the unknown.'
"And he replied,
  'Go out into the darkness and put thine hand into the hand
  of God. That shall be to thee better than light and safer than
  a known way.' "

This parable by M. L. Haskins is a great truth.
If you forget all that you have read in this book,
and if all of it eludes you, go forth and put your
hand in the hand of God — for when you walk with God,
you will always be beautiful . . .

236

Index

1, ch. 1, Will Rogers, ADDRESS, Boston, June, 1930.

2, ch. 1, Alfred Tennyson, ULYSSES, line 18.

1, ch. 2, Channing L. Bete Company, "What Everyone Should Know about Mental Health," Greenfield, Massachusetts, 1980, p.3.

2, ch. 2, Ray Stevens, "Everything Is Beautiful," Nashville, Tennessee, Ray Stevens Music, 1707 Grand Avenue 37212.

3, ch. 2, Jo Tubb, Copley News Service, "There's Cure for Depression," THE WILSON DAILY TIMES, July 3, 1981, p.4c.

4, ch. 2, WORLD BOOK ENCYCLOPEDIA, "Mental Illness," Chicago: Field Enterprises, volume 13, 1978, p. 328.

5, ch. 2, William Henry Drummond, Canadian Poet, 1854-1907. Earlier versions attributed to Etienne (Stephen) de Grellet, 1773-1855.

1, ch. 4, THE WILSON DAILY TIMES. From an article clipped before the book was conceived. Page and date unknown.

2, ch. 4, Louis Harris, THE NEWS AND OBSERVER, November 24, 1978, p.8.

1, ch. 7, Laura Archera Huxley, YOU ARE NOT THE TARGET, New York: Farrar, Strauss, and Giroux, 1973.

1, ch. 8, Ann Landers, THE NEWS AND OBSERVER, February 26, 1981, p.9.

2, ch. 8, Ann Landers, THE NEWS AND OBSERVER, September 4, 1977, p.24, III. Author Unknown.

3, ch. 8, Some attribute the authorship of "I Love You" to Roy Croft. It is often printed as "Author Unknown."

1, ch. 9, Erica Anderson, ALBERT SCHWEITZER'S GIFT OF FRIENDSHIP, New York, Harper and Row, 1964, p.83.

1, ch. 10, Dr. Leo Hawkins, THE WILSON DAILY TIMES, February 7, 1979, p.5.

1, ch. 14, Ann Landers, THE NEWS AND OBSERVER, clipped, no date available.

2, ch. 14, William Shakespeare, MACBETH, Act II, Scene II, line 36.

3, ch. 14, This poem is often reprinted as "Author Unknown" or "Anonymous." However, Wilferd A. Peterson was listed as author on a plaque which gave a part of the poem as a quote.

4, ch. 14, Mental Health Association of Wilson County, Room 619, First Union National Bank, Wilson, North Carolina 27893. Also used by the state organization.

5, ch. 14, Ann Landers, "Who Is Mentally Healthy?" THE NEWS AND OBSERVER, January 18, 1981, III, p.8.

6, ch. 14, "The Courage to Act," Author Unknown. From a quotation in the office of Ambassador Franklin Williams, Washington, D.C., 1971.

1, ch. 15, Ann Landers, THE NEWS AND OBSERVER, October 22, 1978, III, p.17.

2, ch. 15, From THE CONFUCIAN ANALECTS, Book 17:6.

3, ch. 15, William Shakespeare, HENRY THE FIFTH, Act V, Scene II.

1, ch. 23, Dr. Lawrence Lamb, "Health," THE WILSON DAILY TIMES. Clipped. Page number and date not available.

1, ch. 27, Jan Jennings, Copley News Service, THE WILSON DAILY TIMES, December 11, 1980.

1, ch. 28, "Accentuate the Positive," from the movie HERE COME THE WAVES, 1944. Words by Johnny Mercer; music by Harold Arlen.

1, ch. 31, Ann Landers, "Confidential to Hee-Hawed to Death," THE NEWS AND OBSERVER. Clipped. No date available.

1, ch. 35, Shirley Bright Boody, Copley News Service, THE WILSON DAILY TIMES, January 10, 1981, p.78B.

1, ch. 36, United States Department of Agriculture, NUTRITION: FOOD AT WORK FOR YOU, Washington, D.C. 20250, 1978, pp.3, 4.

1, ch. 38, The essays in Part III, written over a period of years, were shared with Tommy Manning, Editor of the Free Will Baptist Press, Ayden, North Carolina, and he published them gratuitously from time to time over a period of years in THE FREE WILL BAPTIST. These essays represent my best thoughts about God and our relationship to Him. Even though a few of the thoughts and quotes are used elsewhere in this book, I hope that the reader will tolerate my leaving the essays intact. JPB

Acknowledgements

My appreciation to the following:

Bob Aiken, Jr., of Snow Hill, N.C., photographer, for reprints of the photograph used on the cover.

Jennie Alexander, reference librarian, Wilson County Public Library, Wilson, N.C., for much patient research.

American Cyanamid Company, Wayne, New Jersey, for permission to recommend Centrum vitamin.

Robert J. Anzelmo, acting assistant head, Publishing Center, Washington, D.C., for permission to quote extensively from publications of the United States Department of Agriculture.

Shirley Bright Boody, of Copley News Service, San Diego, California, for permission to quote from her column, "Eat Yourself Slim," which appears in THE WILSON DAILY TIMES.

Sally R. Cameron, Executive Director of the Mental Health Association of North Carolina, Inc., for permission to use "25 Ways to Brighten Your Days."

Daniel E. Carmody, Director, Educational Services, Channing L. Bete Company, for permission to quote from WHAT EVERYONE SHOULD KNOW ABOUT MENTAL HEALTH.

Helen Clark Collins, of Greenville, N.C., for proofreading.

Jan Davis, of Cary, photographer, for the original photograph that appears on the cover.

Doubleday and Company, 245 Park Avenue, New York, for assistance in tracing quotations.

Theodora Dunkerley and Desmond Dunkerley, Conifers, Heather Lane, High Salvington, Worthing, Sussex, England, for permission to quote "The Ways," by John Oxenham.

The Emporium, of North Hills, Raleigh, N.C., for permission to recommend its products.

Dr. Leo Hawkins, Human Development Specialist, N.C. Agriculture Extension Division, N.C. State University, Raleigh, N.C., for permission to quote extensively from his article, "Listening Is One of the Nicest Things You Do for Children."

Jan Jennings, of the San Diego EVENING TRIBUNE and Copley News Service, for permission to quote from "Choosing the Right Wardrobe Can Give Men, Women, a Competitive Edge," and "How You Dress Matters in the Business World," and other articles quoted from THE WILSON DAILY TIMES.

Johnson and Johnson, New Brunswick, New Jersey, for permission to recommend their products.

Dr. Lawrence E. Lamb, of "The Health Letter," WILSON DAILY TIMES, for permission to quote.

Ann Landers, SUN TIMES, Chicago, Illinois, and Field Newspaper Syndicate, for permission to quote from her column which appears in THE NEWS AND OBSERVER.

Dr. Jack McCall, President, Mental Health Association of North Carolina, for permission to quote him.

Tommy Manning, of San Antonio, Texas, former editor of THE FREE WILL BAPTIST, for permission to reprint editorials which appeared in that magazine.

Kathy Mitchell, of the SUN TIMES, Chicago, for her assistance in obtaining permission to quote from Ann Landers.

Kate Morris, of the Helen Nash Association, Lexington Avenue, New York, for permission to recommend Noxema.

The Pantene Company, Nutley, New Jersey, for permission to recommend its shampoo.

Sam Ragan, Editor, THE PILOT, Southern Pines, for advice and help, especially concerning quotes and copyrights.

John W. Ragsdale, Ray Stevens Music, Grand Avenue, Nashville, Tennessee, for permission to quote from the song, "Everything Is Beautiful."

Dr. W. Burkette Raper, President, Mount Olive College, Mount Olive, North Carolina, for helping to trace "The Courage to Act."

The Rev. Walter Reynolds, Manager, Free Will Baptist Press, Ayden, North Carolina, for permission to reprint my personal editorials which appeared in THE FREE WILL BAPTIST.

Ruth S. Shenker, Consumer Communications Office of Consumer Affairs, Department of Health, Education, and Welfare, Washington, D.C., and Rockville, Maryland, for permission to quote extensively from any materials of that department.

Additional Acknowledgements*

Joseph Addison 20; Louisa Mae Alcott 46; Ambrose 20; James Barrie 17; Alice Bell 28; Bernard Bell 9; Henry Holcomb Bennett 15; John J. Bonica 4; Dr. Herbert Benson 43; Robert Browning 38; Inge Gibson Caldwell 19; Anne Campbell 8; Al Capp 13; Cervantes 9; Chaucer 28; Winston Churchill 16, 33; Cicero 18; Confucius 15; Ernest Crosby 9; Mary Carolyn Davies 6; Austin Dodson 1; Henry Drummond 2; Charles DuBois 50; Katherine Edelman 48; George Eliot 14, 45, 48; Ralph Waldo Emerson 3, 14, 15, 16, 20, 21, 29, 38, 49; Empedocles 9; Epictetus 19; Erasmus 42; Harry Emerson Fosdick 15; Sam Walter Foss 15; Emmet Fox 9; Benjamin Franklin 32, 45; Robert Frost 42; Mahatma Gandhi 15; Arnold H. Glascow 14; J. B. Goode 14; Charles Gordon 38; Billy Graham 39; John Greist 34; Edward Everett Hale 9; John Hare 3; Louis Harris 4; William Henry Harrison 8; M. L. Haskins 54; Helen Hayes 19; Nathaniel Hawthorne 19; William Ernest Henley 15; Heinrich Heine 9; Irene Smith Heyman 19; Holy Bible, King James version 1, 2, 5, 14, 16, 18, 29, 32, 34, 35, 38, 41, 42, 43, 44, 46, 48, 49, 50, 51; Homer 14; Herbert Hoover 8; Victor Hugo 9; John Keats 1; Helen Keller 42; Rudyard Kipling 15, 45; Anne Morrow Lindbergh 18, 19; Abraham Lincoln 19; Henry Wadsworth Longfellow 3, 8, 15, 19; W. J. Lucas 20; Martin Luther 9, 45; Edwin Markham 14; Catherine Marshall 38; Lee Meriwether 17; Joaquin Miller 14; John Milton 14, 42; Napoleon 6; Reinhold Niebuhr 14; Pericles 14; Wilferd A. Peterson 14; Plato 1; Plutarch 14, 20; Alexander Pope 3; Pope John XXIII 3, 4; James Henry Potts 18; John Robert Powers 5; Eugenia Price 41; Helen Steiner Rice 9; Roget's THESAURUS 17; John Ruskin 6;

240

Saint Ambrose 20; Saint Francis of Assisi 9; Carl Sandburg 32; William Shakes-
peare 5, 14; George Bernard Shaw 20; Charlie Shedd 8; Socrates 17; Sophocles 14;
Charles Spurgeon 42; Richard Steele 3; Robert Louis Stevenson 4, 48, 49; Horace
Stewart 14; Muriel Strade 42; Harriet Beecher Stowe 2; Dr. Albert Schweitzer 9;
THE TALMUD 14; Alfred Tennyson 14, 15; William Makepeace Thackeray 14;
Henry David Thoreau 3, 14; John Tillotson 20; Theodore Tilton 14; Leo Tolstoy 9;
Martin Vanbee 29; Marquis de Vauvenargues 3; Webster's SEVENTH NEW
COLLEGIATE DICTIONARY 18; John Wesley 9; John Greenleaf Whittier, 15;
William Wordsworth 9, 48.

*Numbers represent the chapter in which the quotation is found.

Further Acknowledgements

The author and publishers have made every effort to trace the
ownership of all copyrighted material as well as non-copyrighted
information and to indicate proper credit. Should there prove to be
any question, however, regarding the use of any material or information, the author and publishers herewith express regret for such
unconscious error. Upon notification of any error, the publishers will
be pleased to make proper acknowledgement in future editions of this
book.